the
keto
diet

The 60-day plan to transform your health

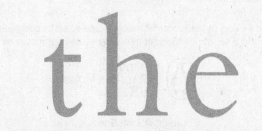

the keto diet

SCOTT GOODING

Vermilion
LONDON

1 3 5 7 9 10 8 6 4 2

Vermilion, an imprint of Ebury Publishing,
20 Vauxhall Bridge Road,
London SW1V 2SA

Vermilion is part of the Penguin Random House group of companies whose
addresses can be found at global.penguinrandomhouse.com

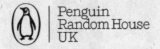

Penguin
Random House
UK

Published in the United Kingdom by Vermilion in 2019

www.penguin.co.uk

A CIP catalogue record for this book is available from the British Library

ISBN 9781785042638

Printed and bound in Great Britain by Clays Ltd, Elcograf S.p.A.

Penguin Random House is committed to a sustainable future for our business,
our readers and our planet. This book is made from Forest Stewardship Council®
certified paper.

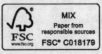

The information in this book has been compiled by way of general guidance in
relation to the specific subjects addressed, but it is not a substitute and not to
be relied on for medical, healthcare, pharmaceutical or other professional advice
on specific circumstances and in specific locations. Please consult your GP before
changing, stopping or starting any medical treatment. So far as the author is
aware the information given is correct and up to date as at December 2018.
Practice, laws and regulations all change, and the reader should obtain up to date
professional advice on any such issue. The author and the publishers disclaim,
as far as the law allows, any liability arising directly or indirectly from the use or
misuse of the information contained in this book.

Contents

Contents

Foreword

I'm a 'pointy head' ... a nerd, a practitioner–researcher ... but I certainly didn't follow a linear path to my current place in the nutrition industry. After being kicked out of high school (a story for another time), I went to university to study fitness, strength training and nutrition. After repeatedly questioning the carb-laden recommendations we were being taught, I was eventually sent to the dean and removed from nutrition class. An inauspicious start in nutrition to be sure, but also one of the best things that ever happened to me. I couldn't reconcile what the science (even all those years ago) was telling us was optimal for the body, and the outdated, highly processed, high-carb dietary recommendations.

From that point on, I became an advocate for a 'carb-appropriate, real-food' approach to nutrition. I achieved amazing results, working with top-level athletes, the morbidly obese and people with chronic health conditions — using lower carb, 'real-food' based interventions. And while I was happy to be helping these clients perform and feel at their very best, it was a lonely existence being out in the wilderness of the nutrition world!

Thankfully, what were fringe areas are now firmly entering the mainstream consciousness and are recognised for their considerable clinical value.

A testament to this shift is that I am now a researcher and PhD candidate in nutrition (specifically in the areas of metabolic adaptation and ketogenesis) at the very same university that kicked me out of nutrition classes for advocating low-carb concepts.

As a practitioner and researcher, I love delving into the science behind nutrition and explaining this science to clients and students, and now, increasingly, answering some of the lingering questions through my research work. But I know as well as anyone that all the science in the world comes to naught if such knowledge can't be applied by real people, in the real world. And that's why I enjoyed reading this book.

Let's face it, we have some challenges. We have increasing rates of metabolic disorder, obesity and diabetes, rapid rises in dementia, Alzheimer's and other neurodegenerative disorders, and cancer and heart disease still take far too many lives. It's clear that our current nutrition environment still isn't serving us well . . .

We're only now beginning to understand the role that metabolic health plays in the development of the major diseases and disorders of the developed world, namely cardiovascular and cerebrovascular diseases, neurodegenerative disorders and cancer. The trend towards obesity, metabolic disorder and diabetes is being mimicked in nearly every country in the world, and these figures are steadily rising despite (misguided) public health initiatives to improve diet and increase activity.

We could even be the very first generation to live a shorter lifespan than our parents despite all the medical advances we've achieved. We're undoing all that good work through poor diet and lifestyle choices. The root of the problem is highly processed, highly refined convenience foods, soft drinks, fruit juice and other added-sugar products. These types of foods don't nourish us sufficiently, don't fill us up, and they don't satisfy us.

I met Scott via mutual acquaintances in the health and nutrition industry. I must say, we hit it off . . . he might even agree! Of course, we share many of the same ideas around health, training and nutrition, but more importantly, I could see that Scott is the 'real deal'. He *walks his talk*. He trains, he moves, he eats *real,* nourishing food, practises mindfulness, and has fun while doing it! And, most importantly, he shares that fun and passion with his clients, readers and fans in a way that they can understand.

The *application* of nutrition is so crucial, as is being empowered on your journey towards optimum health and performance. This empowerment, this connection, shines through in Scott's book, from the motivation for writing the book in Tashi and Eli, through to his own journey in health and wellness.

It's clear in these pages that Scott recognises the value of the whole. He speaks of the interrelated nature of health and wellness and the importance of nutrition, without devaluing other, equally important, aspects of health. And when it comes to the science, he makes it easy to understand without sacrificing validity. Scott presents a positive, empowering and FUN approach to the application of real food, to help you achieve real results, in *your* real life.

I personally took a lot from this book and I know you will too.

Cliff Harvey ND, Dip.Fit, PhD candidate
Author, practitioner and academic researcher in nutrition
Founder of the Holistic Performance Institute
www.cliffharvey.com

Introduction

The reason I do what I do is largely determined by my son, Tashi. *Tashi gives me purpose;* I'm sure this is a feeling most parents can relate to. In this book, I'll be sharing my protocol on the solution to good health – through nutrition and in particular, the benefits of ketosis. We human beings are melting pots of biochemistry, and food is simply 'information' to either positively or negatively influence our health.

My endeavour is to change the current food landscape in the Western world, and Tashi is undoubtedly my number one motivation in this pursuit. I want to see Tashi grow to have better food choices, and for healthy to be the 'norm'.

This book is dedicated to my best friend, Tashi, and to another little boy, Eli. But more about Eli later.

Before I start, I want to flag that along with ketogenesis, there are some quite complex topics covered in this book. Rest assured, however, that I've tried to make them as clear and comprehensible as possible. (I'm no scientist or professor, so to use technical terms would only confuse me!) My goal is to make following a keto diet and all the other information given here as digestible (pun intended) as possible – so simple, in fact, that you'll be able to share what you read tonight with your work colleagues at the water cooler tomorrow. This is information we should *all* grasp and share.

While this book is about transforming your health and lifestyle through a keto diet and in turn a low inflammatory environment, it's worth pointing out that nothing really works in isolation with regards to physiology. Every process affects a myriad of other processes in the body's task of running as efficiently as possible. We are complex, sophisticated, robust and sensitive organisms – products of evolution over millennia – and so you can quickly see that not one thing will work in isolation from another. It's for this reason that I've felt it imperative to cover as much as I can in the simplest possible terms to ensure a broad understanding of the how and the why.

The 'information' in food feeds the biochemistry within us.

Throughout this book, with the exception of Chapter One, I will make a concerted effort not to focus on what has happened in the past and on how the Western world got into a dire health predicament. Nor will I focus on the foods we should reduce, minimise or banish from our lives. Rather, I will focus on moving forward and celebrating living a keto lifestyle and the abundance of foods that *do* allow us to thrive. I hope to communicate to as *many* people as humanly possible – therefore my message needs to be positive, practical and inspiring.

There are *so* many ingredients and foods to celebrate, there's actually little need to talk about the less desirable foods that have been identified in recent years. I believe in making the foods that I *do* embrace look enticing and delicious, and hope to get people's attention that way rather than by harping on about the health risks associated with the other foods.

My protocol embraces real food as the
cornerstone to health.

Okay, back to setting the scene for the rest of the book . . .

If I had to put a number on it, around 80 per cent of good health can be attributed to nutrition, and lifestyle around 20 per cent. With this proportional breakdown in mind, I'll devote the equivalent time/energy for each topic accordingly. With some simple modifications to macronutrients and diet to incorporate ketosis, plus some additional tweaks and hacks, it's very possible to have the summer body you want ALL year around and, much more importantly, be healthy and happy.

I'll break it down into bite-sized chunks (pun intended, once again!) and endeavour to use practical examples wherever possible. I'll introduce you to the concept of ketosis and discuss many related topics — including inflammation, diabetes, brain health, epigenetics and fasting — and will include a heap of keto-friendly recipes to help you on your way to optimal health. My premise is to ensure you're in the best possible position to make informed choices about food, lifestyle and anything that you can control day to day. Knowledge is *power*.

At the very least I hope that this book will be thought-provoking and start discussions (around that water cooler) on ways to maximise health and maximise performance. I want this book to open the proverbial door for you to further explore ways and means to optimise health.

You may read things in the book that you've heard before. Don't see this as a waste of your precious time but as a very necessary step in the process of learning. Hearing or seeing things over and over again helps us to take the new information on board. (Trust me: I have to hear something 146 times before it sinks in!)

PUMPING UP YOUR TYRES

I've been a personal trainer and health coach since 2005, and so for a brief moment I'm going to put the pen down and don my PT hat. This is very necessary before moving on.

Okay, you are now my client and we are about to embark on a keto-led health transformation. We need to discuss a few things before that can take place. First, you need to understand that I'm incredibly optimistic about the future – the future for you and your family – when it comes to optimising health, and that I'm with you 100 per cent of the way. Second, I believe we are *all* capable of being lean and strong and adept, as well as of having great immunity – it's *our natural state*!

Ultimately this book is about learning the most effective and efficient ways to adopt a keto lifestyle and be the best version of yourself. The caveat to this is that there is no magic pill or lotion that gets you there. Rather, it requires discipline and perseverance.

But the reward is the greatest life can offer: health and happiness!

> *By engaging in this diet you'll tap into health, cognitive function and longevity.*

This book is quite clearly about health and, to a lesser extent, the role that fitness plays in that, but as you are now my client I should add that not only do I want you to be healthy but I want you to be *happy*.

INTRODUCING THE 60-DAY KETO PROTOCOL

After many years in the industry, countless hours of reading and researching, plus using my own body as a case study, I've done the hard work for you.

Essentially my protocol is a blend of age-old ideology and emerging strategies to health, in particular new research about the health benefits of ketosis. Much of it will seem familiar and follows commonsense

— but acceptance of and adherence to all aspects of the protocol will bring the most positive change in your health.

It's not radical or extremist . . . because if it were it would be hard to adhere to beyond a few weeks and the book would be called '5 Ways to Shred for Stereosonic!' Instead it's an all-encompassing approach to health, which brings in facets of a keto lifestyle, including macronutrients, micronutrients, exercise, sleep, rest, fasting, hydration and bio-hacking.

Rome wasn't built in a day.

By no means am I suggesting you make ALL the changes overnight, instead, attempt to make small changes over a long period of time for guaranteed success. This book is dedicated to offering an alternative approach to the current health guidelines, guidelines that haven't served us particularly well over the past 60-plus years. To make the transition to a newer and better mindset, I've designed my 60-day Keto Protocol to walk you through the information and present a practical, step-by-step guide.

The protocol includes an introductory week ('On-Ramp'), which is the perfect opportunity to set you up for the forthcoming weeks and the best possible position for success. The 60-day Keto Protocol will help reduce inflammation through diet and lifestyle and amplify health. The prerequisite is that you adhere to the programme 100 per cent — to achieve the maximum physiological change and fat adaptation.

My solution, or protocol, is easy to follow and understand — I've shared over 100 recipes to help you on your way. By following my recommendations, you'll be well on your way to optimising your health and happiness. So, sit back, grab some activated nuts and enjoy the journey.

PART ONE

Understanding Keto

Chapter One

Real food

One of my non-negotiables in life is to constantly educate myself and expand my mind. I do this through study, workshops, books, YouTube and podcasts. It's important to grow, learn and evolve, otherwise I'd be nothing more than a piece of granite. This constant evolution is no more apparent than when I look back at my message as a personal trainer over a decade ago. Back in 2005, I thought the solution to all the world's problems was to prescribe cardiovascular exercise. Even my business card stated 'Specialist in Aerobic Conditioning'. The importance of *nutrition* didn't carry the weight that it does for me today.

I dare say that my message and philosophy will continue to refine and evolve in accordance with new research, but as I write this today, I firmly believe that exercise is not the solution to health and weight management. For decades we have made fitness, exercise and working out the marker of health and the solution to weight loss. I understand that I might be talking myself out a job, but the first thing we should do is accept and understand that we can be healthy, lean and have a strong immunity from nutrition alone. Now don't throw out those tatty gym shoes just yet — I'm not suggesting that fitness hasn't a role to play; it most certainly does. I'm merely suggesting we can afford to relieve ourselves of the guilt if we miss a day, a week or a month of training and instead redirect our time and energy into making our nutrition the solution to health.

OKAY, SO THINGS ARE LOOKING UP, RIGHT?

You can relax a little, safe in the knowledge I'm not about to prescribe burpees (a hideous exercise designed by the devil himself!), hill sprints or star jumps . . . for the time being, anyway! So if training isn't the Holy Grail, what is? Well, if I told you that your great-grandma had the answer, you'd probably look bemused. I'd like you to meet *my* great-grandma, Jean. Three generations older than me (and, important to note, very much alive and kicking in my lifetime), Jean was the queen of her home. Incredibly resourceful, she spent much of her day creating food for her family. It was an era when food and mealtimes were the focus of home life. Jean made everything from scratch. Most was grown in her back garden, and anything not home-grown was sourced from the local markets. It's safe to say that Jean cooked with local, organic, *real* food. If we were to join Jean for dinner — and this could be any day of the week — we'd be served up meat and three veg, guaranteed.

If we dug a little deeper, we'd see that Jean had no reservations about cooking with the much-maligned saturated fats — butter, ghee, beef dripping, lard and duck fat, to name a few . . . and damn did it taste *good*! In addition, Jean didn't rely on refined, processed food — it barely existed back then — just simple produce cooked with love.

SO WHAT'S THE TAKE-HOME MESSAGE HERE?

It's pretty straightforward . . . let's get back in touch with the way Jean did things in the kitchen. I'm not suggesting a séance or ouija board, but more along the lines of adopting Jean's staple principles around using *real food*. Jean's cooking was simple, familiar, comfortable and nourishing, for a number of reasons. Great-grandma Jean stuck to the following rules:

1. Eat real food
2. Use saturated fats
3. Have veggies with every meal
4. Eat meals full of flavour

It's worth noting that Jean wasn't cooking for health. Instead, she cooked with produce that she could afford and that was available. Despite her focus not being on health, she actually ticked all the boxes for me. Meal after meal, her creations would be reminiscent of the dishes that I'd happily serve up today – dishes full of healthful, delicious ingredients.

The question has to be asked: how, in the space of just three generations, did we arrive at the food landscape we see today in the Western world?

SWEET, SWEET SUGAR

Sugar in its various guises is the common ingredient found in most of the food items that line our supermarket aisles. How sugar went from obscurity to king status makes for fairly interesting reading.

For a long time, the mechanism for obesity and diabetes was little understood. Obesity was attributed to gluttony and a lack of willpower, but then, prior to World War II, Austrian and German scientists began to reveal that there was more to the picture. Rather than simply the consequence of eating too much, they suggested that obesity could be a hormonal condition, linked to genetics, metabolism and the endocrine system. Just as more support for this theory was gaining traction, the war started, which abruptly halted further research. It wasn't until the late 1950s and 1960s that the conversation was picked up again and science began to talk about the hormone insulin (significant in diabetes) and the fact that insulin could be the driver for obesity . . . and that sugar was a dominant driver of insulin.

In response to this, *artificial sugars* began to rise in popularity as a solution to using real sugar. But the sugar industry was quick to extinguish any threat to its economy. It funded studies to show that artificial sugars were inherently bad for our health, and so paved the way for global dominance.

The conversation flared up again the next decade. In the 1970s, British nutritionist John Yudkin suggested that it *was* sugar that was the bad guy when it came to obesity and diabetes. This again rattled the sugar industry, which responded by funding a campaign that would suggest that saturated fat was the cause of obesity and diabetes, and ultimately divert attention from the real culprit: sugar.

At this point in time it was pretty easy to convince the public, the Food and Drug Administration (FDA) and the government, since in 1958 Ancel Keyes, an American nutritionist, had single-handedly persuaded the US that saturated fat increased cholesterol, which he proposed was the link to coronary heart disease. His study ('The Seven Countries Study') had simply cherry-picked seven out of the 22 countries whose data aligned with his hypothesis. This epidemiological study, which would lack credibility by today's testing standards, was enough to get saturated fats over the line and begin the shift in attitude that is still being felt today, 60 years later.

SUGAR GETS THE GREEN LIGHT

The vilification of saturated fat had left the door wide open for sugar, and so sugar boldly began its journey to global dominance, unhindered and unthreatened. Since the 1960s, we've lapped up sugar with gusto. You only have to meander through your local supermarket or food court to gain an understanding of how sugar is the dominant ingredient. Pretty much every processed food item will feature sugar to a greater or lesser extent, and let's not forget that refined carbs (bread, cereals, pasta) have the same hormonal response as sugar — but more on this shortly. If we knew the health implications of consuming too much sugar decades ago, why didn't we put the brakes on? To me the answer is multilayered, but two important reasons to consider are:

1. It's not me, it's my hormones

As *Homo sapiens* we are genetically geared to consume sugar. Let's go back a few score millennia (even before Great-grandma Jean!) and observe how hunter–gatherers consumed sugar. Their access to sugar was seasonal, not perennial, for they found it mostly in the form of fruits. When it was available they would simply gorge on it. It's the law of optimal foraging: get as many calories in, in the most efficient way, in order to preserve energy. Maximising intake of food was an important strategy, as the 'cupboard' could be bare tomorrow.

To prepare for leaner times, our body triggers a hormonal response to ensure we come back to the hunter–gatherer cookie jar. (Anyone who has polished off an entire jar of Nutella in one sitting knows what I'm talking about — it's not *you*, it's your hormones.)

When we consume sugar, receptors on our tongue send a signal to the brain stem and from there it branches off to the forebrain and a specialised part of the brain called the cerebral cortex. This area of the brain recognises different taste sensations: bitter, sweet, salty, sour, etc. Now (this is the important thing to wrap our heads around), from here a message is sent to activate our brain's reward system, which is a series of electrical and chemical pathways. This process is incredibly complex but it helps to answer one inner thought: 'Should I have another bite of the doughnut?' The answer is invariably a resounding YES, because you feel all warm and fuzzy . . . and let's be honest, who doesn't like to feel warm and fuzzy! (Note that this reward system isn't only activated by sugar but by other, finer things in life, like socialising and sex . . . so again, it's not *you*, it's your hormones!) The currency for this reward system is a neurotransmitter called dopamine, and dopamine is the reason we come back for more and more.

Over-activating the dopamine reward system can lead to increased tolerance to sugar, as well as to cravings, and much like drugs such as alcohol, nicotine and cocaine that also trigger dopamine, we come back for more . . . and it's not long before we have an addiction.

Sugar is in fact regarded as seven or eight times more addictive than cocaine. In a study at Princeton University, 43 rats were offered cocaine or sugar water over a 15-day period. Forty of the 43 trial rats preferred the sugar water. In a similar experiment, rats exhibited eating behaviours such as binging, craving and withdrawals when on a high-sugar diet. Admittedly, studies of this nature aren't as well verified on humans — it's most likely the combination of sugar *and* fat *and* sodium that is the addictive recipe in the Western diet.

2. Strip fat and you strip mouth-feel and taste

Once saturated fat was outlawed and marched to the proverbial county border back in the 1960s, it gave birth to the age of *low-fat*. I remember growing up being surrounded by advertising about skimmed this, low-fat that . . . a message that was pushed so hard for so long that it's now entrenched in our food landscape and influences our spend at the supermarket. But going from full-fat to low-fat or fat-reduced products presented manufacturers with a conundrum: how were they to replace the mouth-feel and taste that fat provides?

The answer was simple: sugar. Sugar was a cheap commodity, and manufacturers knew we loved it, so overnight low-fat products such as yoghurt were pumped full of sugar. From an industry point of view, this was a stroke of genius. It was like a drug-dealer giving someone their first shot of heroin — they knew they'd come back for more.

But let's get back to the task at hand . . .

Remember how I want you to be the healthiest and happiest person you can be? As my client, it is my duty of care to provide you with the easiest, safest path to achieving this goal.

SO, WHAT'S FIRST?

There is little sense in bio-hacking and fine-tuning your health if the foundation isn't dealt with appropriately. It's like an architect paying all his/her attention on the ornate details of the house when the structure is fundamentally flawed . . . it just doesn't make sense!

With this in mind, we'll work on the foundation of health: nutrition. I firmly believe it's our genetic blueprint to be lean, strong, have good immunity and longevity — and that this can be achieved through nutrition. The version of nutrition that I'm promoting may be slightly different to that which we have become accustomed to in the Western world, but bear with me. I'm not interested in a quick-fix solution for health or weight loss; I'm interested in the adoption of a new lifestyle.

FIRST STEP: REAL FOOD

Real food is simply better for you! Let's define real food. It's *food in its most natural state, either grown in the ground, on a bush or on a tree, or that was once an animal or derived from one.* You get the picture? In essence, real food is food which resembles what it was in its natural state, with no added nasties.

Real food served Great-grandma Jean and countless generations before her well, and will serve us well as we move forward. We just have to navigate the food landscape a little harder in order to find it. *Real food* is more than just calories; it provides important 'information' — information that our bodies use in order to send signals, elicit certain hormones and influence which genes are turned on or off. The topic of nutrition and its many health ramifications is incredibly broad, so I'll aim to tackle this over a few chapters. For now, the key take-home message is that *real food* is more nutrient dense than refined food. The time to demonise refined, processed foods has passed; the time to celebrate and embrace real foods is upon us. *Real food* will have macronutrients (fats, proteins and carbohydrates) as well as possess the micronutrients necessary for function and health. A lack of essential micronutrients is often the cause for sub-optimal health and even disease.

Eating *real food* will ensure you're getting your vitamins and minerals from a rich and varied source – the more varied the better. Our early ancestors utilised hundreds of food sources, including herbs, spices, flowers, nuts, seeds, insects, game and fish. It's reasonable to surmise that the majority of Westerners today receive the bulk of their nutrients from just a handful of food groups, based on diet-related health epidemics. It makes sense to get your nutrients from as many sources as possible. Insufficient intake of vitamins can lead to conditions such as scurvy and rickets, experienced in the past by sailors whose diets consisted of non-perishable foods such as biscuits and oats, which lacked essential vitamins and minerals.

There are plenty of examples of how *real food* has provided therapeutic assistance and reduced the symptoms of specific conditions, but we can go a step further and talk about *real food* being downright medicinal, and how it can *reverse* conditions and bring unwell people back to good health.

In 2000, physician Terry Wahls was diagnosed with multiple sclerosis, for which there is no conventional cure. This condition is one that is close to my heart, as my uncle and nan suffered for many years with it. Dr Wahls sought the best treatment she could find, but by 2003 her condition had worsened to secondary progressive MS. Prior to diagnosis, Dr Wahls was a tae kwon do champion, but soon she found herself relying on a wheelchair. Appalled with her decline in health, Dr Wahls embarked on a strategy outside of the conventions of Western medicine. Using herself as a guinea pig, she identified certain symptoms that were common amongst MS, Alzheimer's and Parkinson's sufferers and hatched a plan on how to combat them. It took her down a path of supplements in the form of vitamins and minerals. Immediately, she witnessed a slowing of her condition but decided to take it a step further. Rather than relying on store-bought supplements, she attempted to replace these with *real food,* acknowledging that *real food* would not only provide therapeutic properties for her MS but supply a heap of other 'information' which might benefit her.

Over time, her symptoms slowed and eventually reversed. Her mobility returned.

Taking a clinical approach to her diet, Dr Wahls unveiled what was to become her 'protocol' — a system of rules which would eventually help thousands of people around the world. Her personal focus was on optimal health and ensuring she took in sufficient information (co-factors) through *real food* to provide the building blocks for trillions of chemical reactions within her body, thus setting herself up for great health.

I'm not suggesting we get clinical about our food; in fact, quite the opposite — food still needs to be enjoyed. But having a fundamental understanding of what *is* and what *isn't* good for us is a simple strategy for ensuring that your body gets enough of the good stuff.

Dr Wahls suggests your daily intake include:

3 cups of green leaves   Greens such as spinach and kale are rich in vitamins B, C, K and A and can be added to make your morning smoothie more nutrient-dense. Other leafy greens include Swiss chard, spring greens, turnip greens, red and green leaf and Romaine lettuce, cabbage, pak choi and watercress.

3 cups of sulphur-rich veggies   Cruciferous veggies are rich in sulphur, which is incredibly important for liver and kidney function and is instrumental in removing toxins from the bloodstream. Examples of sulphur-rich vegetables are cabbage, Brussels sprouts, broccoli, cauliflower, rocket, radish, turnip, onions, garlic, leeks and mushrooms.

3 cups of bright colour   This can be a combination of veggies and fruit and should include pumpkin, carrot, beetroot and berries.

Dr Wahls's protocol also includes other food groups, which I'll touch on later in this book, but knowing that there are things growing in the ground that can allow us to thrive and support our entire system is valuable knowledge.

BUT VEGGIES ARE BORING!

Not everything that is healthy tastes exciting, right, especially if you're comparing salted caramel Häagen-Dazs to steamed broccoli. Knowing that cabbage, for instance, is healthy doesn't automatically mean we'll chow down on a whole bowl of it. If that was the case, I'm confident I wouldn't be writing this book! It would be great if we all craved Brussels sprouts and kale, but sadly our hormones aren't working for us in this respect. A bowl of broccoli doesn't set our world alight or trigger significant levels of dopamine in our reward centre, so we have to work a little harder to make veggies the hero of the day.

So, what are some really simple ways to make the humble veggie more glamorous?

1. Add healthy fats

Adding fat to your veggies will not only increase their nutrient density but will add some crucial flavour. Try adding some butter or ghee to warmed veggies (butter makes *everything* taste better, for the record!) or some decent extra-virgin olive oil. Alternatively, you could throw on some nut oil such as walnut or macadamia. Having a few different fats/oils at hand means you can begin to be more nuanced in adding taste.

Add a fat to the cooking process, too. Animal fats such as lard, beef dripping and duck fat are great for adding flavour and studies have shown that cooking with olive oil, for example, can increase the yield of antioxidants. In other words, antioxidants can migrate or transfer from the oil to the veggies. Interesting stuff!

2. Add lemon

The humble lemon is a staple in my kitchen, and when I'm not making lemon meringue pie (eye roll) I'm squeezing it on my salad, my lamb, my steak and my avocado. It has the ability to lift most dishes and is an affordable way to brighten your veggies.

3. Add salt

Any chef will tell you, season your food. In fact, I learned of the importance of seasoning through my experience on a cooking show, *My Kitchen Rules*. During the early stages of the competition I was criticised for under-seasoning. Ironically, I was booted out in the semi-finals for over-seasoning! Do make sure it is a good salt, though — simple sea salt and Himalayan pink salt are both rich in minerals.

4. Cook quickly

Please don't cook the life out of your veggies — no-one likes grey, overcooked broccoli! Overcooking will deplete the veggies' nutrient stockpile, so look to lightly sauté your greens (include the stems, too, for added nutrients and prebiotics — more on this later). Resist exposing vegetables to high heat; they'll respond better to a low/medium heat. And remove them from the heat as soon as they begin to soften. The residual heat will further cook them. Aim to have a little crunch in your cooked veg.

5. Add chilli

Not everyone's cup of tea, but if you are a fan of spice, adding some dried, crushed or fresh chilli can add some sexiness. Chillies are also powerful anti-inflammatories.

6. Add a dressing

Even the most bland veggie (yes, I'm talking to you, Mr Courgette) can be transformed by adding a dressing. This can be as simple as a vinaigrette, olive oil and lemon juice, a tahini dressing or a nuoc cham (Asian dipping sauce).

7. Use one or more of the above

The bottom line is to make veggies sexy and delicious, so do whatever is necessary to make them enticing to you and your family. And remember to mix things up. Don't cook the same veggies day in day out, otherwise you'll get bored and drop them altogether. The more exciting you make veggies and the more often you make them exciting, the more they will ignite your dopamine, giving you that warm and fuzzy feeling when you eat something delicious.

There isn't one diet on this planet — well, not one I've come across anyway — that advocates eating fewer veggies. So, let's shout about them from the rooftops! Make them shiny, glittery and delicious and you'll be ticking a HUGE health box. As an architect of your own health, eating a broad range of veggies is setting some really solid foundations — so start building today!

Chapter Two

Low inflammation is key

One of the cornerstone messages of this book concerns inflammation. For the last decade or so I've talked about diet and nutrition, and at times attached a label to it, whether it's 'paleo diet', 'ancestral health' or 'primal diet', but when you strip it back it's all about inflammation.

As your health coach, please listen as I tell you that minimising inflammation is pivotal to health. If you trace any health condition or disease back to its root, you'll discover that it is due to inflammation, so let's unpack this a little more so we are all on the same page. *Everything* will make sense from here on in.

My approach is not just high fat/low carb, but nutrition that promotes a low-inflammatory internal environment. To grasp this notion we have to look at our digestive tract — not the sexiest part of the anatomy, but arguably the most important. Let's go on a little trip down your digestive tract. (For anyone old enough to remember the film *Innerspace*, this is a good reference point.)

Several times a day we shove food and drinks in our mouth, and we've done this nearly every single day of our lives — but what happens?

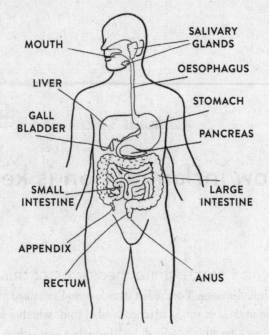

MOUTH — SALIVARY GLANDS

LIVER — OESOPHAGUS

GALL BLADDER — STOMACH

— PANCREAS

SMALL INTESTINE — LARGE INTESTINE

APPENDIX

RECTUM — ANUS

MOUTH

Digestion begins here and works on a couple of levels. Mechanical action on the food helps to break the food down in size, which increases its surface area, making it easier to digest and absorb nutrients. Simultaneously, the saliva glands release saliva, mucus and enzymes to further digest the food particles.

OESOPHAGUS

Once we swallow, wave-like muscular contractions push the food down the oesophagus. Where the oesophagus meets the stomach there is a valve that prevents stomach acid entering the oesophagus.

STOMACH

Your stomach is a highly acidic environment with a pH of 1.5 to 3.5. This acidity helps to break down food and will also kill any pathogens. A heap of enzymatic reactions break down the food to a semi-fluid mass called chyme.

SMALL INTESTINE

This is the site where most of the digestion takes place. On the wall of the small intestine, there are finger-like projections that serve to increase surface area and in order to provide maximum absorbency of nutrients. It's the absorbency of nutrients that is crucial to our health. 'We are what we eat'? Hmmm, nearly! **'We are what we *absorb*'.**

LARGE INTESTINE

Any matter that evades digestion in the small intestine is then passed through to the large intestine. Insoluble fibre or resistant starches are good examples of what might be found here. It's in our large intestine that our microbiome live. Trillions of bacteria (good and bad) live in a diverse environment. There are more bacteria in our gut than cells in our entire body! Faeces are produced in our large intestine, ready to be passed through to the anus as stools.

ANUS

The anus is the last part of the digestive tract and its function is to control the expulsion of faeces. In healthy individuals, stools are soft and easy to pass. Incidentally, the colour of stools has less to do with the foods consumed than with the removal of dead blood cells and the level of hydration in the body.

Throughout the entire digestive process, trillions of chemical reactions occur to ensure we absorb all the 'information' the food contains. It's this information that sets us up for health or ill-health.

Let's backtrack up the digestive tract a little (a horrid thought!) and chat about the significance of the large intestine some more. You may have heard of the terms microbiome, or gut flora, or good and bad bacteria — well, this is where they reside. This area of the body has been studied for decades but it's only really in the last five or six years that we have really begun to grasp the role and significance of the gut.

It's a dark, noisy, thriving, bustling rainforest with more life than you'd believe. I often think we are simply a vehicle for our bacteria, as it's them that decide our moods, our cravings, our immunity and much, much more. It's an odd concept to grasp, but delve into this area and you'll begin to understand what I mean. It is the condition of our microbiome that will largely determine our health — both physically and mentally. Hence it's imperative that we foster a healthy microbiome. But what does that even mean?

As I've just described, the significance of the gut cannot be overlooked. In broad terms, most of our serotonin is manufactured in our gut, most of our immunity is made in our gut, and a nerve (the vagus nerve) links directly between the gut and the brain. (See, I told you nothing works in isolation!)

The importance of your gut health is the reason I'm not prescribing push-ups and burpees. *This* is the Holy Grail to health. Do as many squats and push-ups as you like, *but*, if your gut is sub-optimal, you'll be spinning your wheels. Spend your time and energy nurturing and fostering a happy gut environment and you'll be the happiest, shiniest version of yourself.

The beautiful thing is, no matter how much you've abused your body and consequently your gut over the years, you can still make good. It's simply a case of dialling back or amplifying certain foods and lifestyle choices.

I once heard the amazing Robb Wolf say that as long as we are above the ground, we have the ability to influence our health in a positive way and be the best version of ourselves. I absolutely love this notion. Too many of us are content with our 'lot', but we can all strive for great health and happiness, and once you've had a taste of it, you won't want anything less.

Let's have a look at the factors that will influence your gut health for the good and the bad.

THE GOOD

Vaginal birth

This is obviously not something you had any say in, but it's of interest to know that being born vaginally gives your gut an upfront advantage. In utero, a baby has very little gut flora and receives all its nutrients from its mother through the umbilical cord. During its passage down the vaginal canal, however, a baby is exposed to anal and vaginal fluids. It's all completely natural and necessary, and provides microbes to the emerging baby. It's during this process that the baby lays down the foundation of its gut microbiome.

Caesarean birth (C-section), which is on the rise in the Western world, obviously bypasses this delivery route and baby misses out on the transference of vaginal and faecal matter (bacteria) from the mum. It goes without saying that C-section is necessary in some cases — and thankfully there are strategies that ensure that the baby receives microbes from its mother during C-section. Ask your midwife or obstetrician about them.

If the baby is breastfed, it's also given a bunch of new bacteria.

Diverse bacteria

We live in a sanitised world and are told to fear bacteria, but having the *right* bacteria in the *right* place is in fact incredibly important. Just as we should endeavour to get our nutrients from a broad variety of foods, the same applies for bacteria. Eating *real food* is one way of exposing ourselves to a broad variety of bacteria. Another is to get our hands dirty – quite literally. Many of us, particularly us city-dwellers, lack exposure to land-based bacteria. We simply don't get our hands in the earth these days and so miss out on a bunch of bacteria. Kids growing up in rural areas, particularly around animals, have a different and diverse microbiome compared to their city counterparts.

The Hadza tribe, one of the few remaining hunter–gatherer tribes in the world, from northern Tanzania, have amongst the most diverse microbiome in the world. Their diet is incredibly varied and includes porcupine, tubers, wild berries and zebra. They've lived this lifestyle for around 40,000 years. Dr Tim Spector, Professor of Genetic Epidemiology at King's College, London, spent time with the Hadza tribe and ate what they ate, and after just three days the diversity of bacteria in his already healthy microbiome had increased by 20 per cent.

Faecal transplant

Sounds hideous, I know, and please don't try this at home, but transplanting faecal matter from a healthy individual into the colon of someone with a health condition can radically alter the gut community of the recipient and lessen, or even reverse, symptoms. Trials of faecal transplant have been used to treat ulcerative colitis, Crohn's disease, IBS, constipation, auto-immune disorders, obesity, Parkinson's disease, multiple sclerosis, chronic fatigue, anxiety and depression.

Fermented foods

Fermented foods such as kimchi, kefir and sauerkraut have become popular in recent years but have been a method of preserving foods for centuries. Fermented foods provide valuable organisms or probiotics. If they aren't already on your radar, start looking out for them, or consider making them yourself. If you're buying fermented foods, be sure to grab products that haven't been pasteurised, otherwise you're wasting your time . . . and money!

The microbes found in fermented food are heavyweights, resistant to digestion in the stomach and small intestine simply because they have grown in an acidic environment. Therefore, by the time they reach the large intestine, they are able to make themselves at home.

Prebiotics

Prebiotics are foods that survive digestion in the small intestine and provide 'food' for the bacteria in the large intestine. Sources of prebiotics include onion, garlic, asparagus, Jerusalem artichokes, lentils and beans. Green bananas also contain helpful gut-feeding elements, but as they ripen the sugar content begins to skyrocket, so get in early and they'll serve you as prebiotics.

Prebiotic foods are broken down in an anaerobic environment to produce methane. This is an explanation for the wind produced by the abovementioned foods. So it's not *you*, it's your bacteria! (I always blame the dog, anyway.)

THE BAD

Antibiotics

As a means of combating bacterial infections, antibiotics are the common solution. A course of antibiotics not only attacks the offending bacteria but acts like a carpet bomb, eradicating both the harmful and the all-important good bacteria. The fall-out from a round of antibiotics is that it can take up to 12 months to rejuvenate the gut community that it destroyed. Antibiotics certainly have their place, but be mindful of the impact they have on our microbes.

Sanitation and hygiene

You've heard the commercials on the TV proclaiming that this or that spray eradicates 99.9 per cent of germs . . . but is that a particularly good thing?

In a bid to live in a clean world, we have arguably compromised our immunity and gut community. Sprays and hand wipes halt the transference of beneficial microbes. Even the 'yucky' microbes serve a purpose in this equation.

A microbe, upon entering our body, is recognised by our immune system as an invader, eliciting an immune response. The body has a clear understanding of what is foreign and what is not. When everything is sanitised, however, the distinction is not so clear, and so either the body overreacts to invaders as the immune system goes into hyper-drive, or the body attacks itself, as in the case with auto-immune diseases.

The bottom line is, let your kids play in the dirt, and do a spot of gardening every now and then.

Alcohol

Sorry to be the bearer of bad news but alcohol is on this list — not really surprising, is it? Aside from improving your ability to dance, there are few things that alcohol is good for, physiologically. Having been raised in a pub, I'm very familiar with booze. I still choose to drink, but the occasions on which I do are getting fewer and fewer. The odd glass of wine every now and then does allow me to 'switch off' — which, for someone like me, is beneficial. But, yes, booze disrupts the digestive tract by causing inflammation.

Processed foods

I'm sure you're not surprised to find junk food on this list. Just like *real food* contains 'information' (in this case, information to help us thrive), so does junk food . . . just not the kind our body needs. Processed foods come with a bunch of synthetic compounds that irritate the gut and cause distress and inflammation. Couple that with some of the immunogenic foods (ones that elicit an immune response) and we are setting ourselves up for systemic inflammation, which is far from ideal. More on this shortly.

RESISTANT STARCH AND THE GUT

Essentially, resistant starch is, as its name suggests, starch that avoids digestion in the small intestine, but instead proceeds further down the digestive tract to the large intestine (colon). It's in the large intestine that resistant starches become valuable food for our gut microbes. It's imperative that we foster a healthy gut environment and part of that equation involves 'feeding' our gut – see it as feeding your internal pet.

Eating more veggies will help to 'feed' the gut. The microbes in your gut *love* resistant starch, so start to consider cooking and eating the stalks of veggies, such as chard and broccoli. Foods high in resistant starch also include green banana, Jerusalem artichoke, garlic, onion, peas and lentils. Generally speaking, a diet in refined foods will deliver low resistant starch, compared with a 'real-food' diet. Remember that real food contains FAR more 'information' and part of this information is designed to feed your internal pet. If you are striving for nine cups of veggies per day, you'll be well on your way to increasing your resistant starch levels. However, I'd recommend going that extra mile to ensure your pet is content and well fed. A little caveat at this point – if you decide to consume vast quantities of resistant starch tomorrow, after years of it not being on your landscape, then expect to experience some discomfort, bloating and wind. This is all completely normal but try to introduce a little at a time and increase your intake as your body adjusts.

Our gut community is a wild, hostile environment where it's every microbe for itself. Each microbe (and there are hundreds of trillions of them) has its own set of needs and competes against other microbes for dominance.

The gut is much more than where your food is digested. It contains more microbes than the number of people that have ever walked on this planet or the number of cells in your body. Each one of us has a unique gut community, as a direct result of diet, lifestyle, stress, exposure to land-based microbes, method of birth, genetics and so on. With each microbe having its own agenda and needs, it's fair to make the assumption that there is no one diet that fits all – it just doesn't work that way. Based on the diversity and ratios of microbes within an individual, one person will be able to tolerate certain foods better than another person. You might witness this within your family or within your circle of friends. This notion that not one diet fits all is called bio-individuality.

That being said, there are many similarities and commonalities between us. For one thing, no-one thrives on junk food, just as no-one thrives from smoking cigarettes – on this we can all agree.

I mentioned that the route to ill-health is inflammation, so let's explore this a little before looking at practical tools and solutions.

We are all familiar with the mechanism of inflammation on some level. When you stub your toe, your brain receives signals from the area of trauma and sets about a treatment plan: it sends an immune response to first protect the wound from further damage, then to repair disrupted tissues – hence the change in colour and swelling. This type of inflammation is easy to see and understand, but when it comes to inflammation that causes general ill-health, we are referring to a type that isn't visible and is systemic rather than localised. This makes it harder to diagnose and ultimately intervene. It's imperative to minimise systemic inflammation.

The types of food we consume have a huge impact on our gut and the integrity of the gut wall. When things are all working in harmony, the immune cells within our gut are kept from our bacteria. The thing that keeps them separate is the gut lining, and in particular a viscous, snot-like substance called mucin. The production of mucin requires energy in the form of short-chain fatty acids, which can be derived from the breakdown of resistant starches (asparagus and Jerusalem artichoke, etc.). If, however, these are lacking in your diet and there's a heavier reliance on refined foods and sugar, then this ultimately compromises the production of mucin.

What happens next is scary — grab your security blanket!

With a weak barrier between the immune cells and bacteria, the immune cells attack the bacteria and produce what's called an endotoxin. This endotoxin then crosses the gut lining and enters the bloodstream and . . .

But wait. Before I go into the consequence of this, we have to quickly visit the role of cholesterol in the body. (As I've mentioned, nothing works in isolation!)

CHOLESTEROL

Where to start with this guy? Poor ol' cholesterol has endured a tough time over recent years and has been blamed for coronary heart disease, strokes and high blood pressure, but for the time being let's leave the stigma to one side and focus on the positive role that cholesterol plays.

The first thing we need to acknowledge is that every cell in our body (that's *every* cell!) requires cholesterol; it's imperative for cell function and is part of the cell membrane. Most of your cholesterol is manufactured in your liver, and it's a lipoprotein — specifically, a low-density lipoprotein (LDL) — that transports cholesterol *from* the liver to cells around your body. Consider LDL like an Uber driver for your cholesterol, carrying fats wherever they're required or stored. Cells that are being created, need repair or are inflamed will have LDL drop off some cholesterol at the cell site. Because it has donated some cholesterol to the site, it is now considered *small* LDL. In a perfect world the small LDL drives back to the liver, where it parks and comes out of circulation (the bloodstream).

THERE'S TROUBLE BREWING . . .

So if your diet and lifestyle haven't been ideal and have left your gut lining compromised, your endotoxins attach themselves to the floating small LDL that are returning to your liver. But these little suckers actually attach to the docking site on the small LDL, meaning that when it returns to the liver it's unable to dock and be taken out of circulation.

Now this floating cocktail of small LDL and endotoxins sets off alarm bells for the immune system, and action is taken to 'kill' the perceived foreign invader. But action *isn't* taken, for it's not a live bacteria and the immune system isn't sure how to extinguish the threat. Instead, it calls for back-up and in no time the small LDL becomes a cluster of cholesterol, endotoxins and immune cells, otherwise known as a plague. This is problematic! The cluster — a small, dense lipoprotein — is a marker for specific health conditions.

BUT WAIT, THERE'S MORE . . .

When the body has been subject to long-term exposure to poor food or lifestyle choices, the gut lining stops being a robust barrier and starts to look more like a pair of fishnet stockings. Now don't get me wrong, I'm a fan of fishnet stockings, but not in this instance!

The gut lining is designed to serve us in a way that fuels optimal health — remember, our body's primary aim is survival, so when everything is in order things run smoothly. The harmony between our microbes, our gut and our health is only attained when we eat the right foods and minimise other disruptive factors. The factors that affect this harmony include poor nutrition, sleep, external stress, antibiotics and birth history. It's impossible to alter your birth history (vaginal versus C-section) until we invent time travel — but we can control or influence the other factors to promote a healthy gut environment.

Consider the cells within your gut lining to be a long line of workers that stand shoulder to shoulder and create an impenetrable barrier between the gut and the peripheral system (blood). Their role is to absorb nutrients and vitamins (food) from the gut and pass them into the bloodstream – they do this at their own rate and are selective as to what they pass through. When certain factors negatively influence the integrity of the gut lining, the workers are no longer standing shoulder to shoulder and the barrier is compromised. Now the cells' ability to absorb nutrients, as well as prevent the contents of the gut, including undigested food particles, to cross the lining and penetrate the peripheral system (blood), is impaired: the workers cannot control what is transferred and at what rate. This is a condition called 'leaky gut', and can cause an immune response that leads to inflammation, just like the endotoxins.

As I've mentioned, there are many factors that contribute to increased gut permeability and ideally we should aim to minimise them as much as we can. However, it's important to be realistic and acknowledge that eating well, having optimal sleep and generally skipping through life isn't achievable every single day. At this stage it's simply important to understand the mechanisms for leaky gut.

One of the factors that directly affects our health is sleep – the importance of sleep cannot be overlooked or underestimated. Having poor sleep can lead to increased desire for poor foods, foods that compromise your gut lining. Throw external stress in the mix too and you have a familiar yet sub-optimal situation. I bet you can name plenty of people who are stressed out and have poor sleep – this combination affects hormones and our desire for sugary foods/drinks increases. A diet high in sugary foods affects the harmony of our gut balance, ultimately affecting our own ability to produce mucin, the snot-like substance that acts like a mucous barrier for our gut lining.

The deep importance of sleep to our health was exemplified by a recent study by Dr Eran Elinav, an expert in the relationship between the immune system, intestinal microbiota and health and disease.

Subjects of the study flew across different time zones to induce jet-lag and the stress associated with it. Faecal samples from the subjects were then placed into healthy mice. The results were astonishing. The mice who received microbes from the jet-lagged students grew obese and developed diabetes; mice that received microbes from students not exposed to jet-lag saw no change — mind blowing!

As I have stated, the cornerstone to ill-health or disease is systemic inflammation. Since a compromised gut lining is a major contributor to inflammation, I strongly recommend introducing some tricks and hacks that promote a happy gut environment. Start by cherishing sleep — nothing feels better than getting an early night — introducing some prebiotics (resistant starch) and maximising 'information-rich' food — real food!

Certain foods, such as grains, dairy and legumes (broadly speaking), can cause irritation to the gut lining due to the foods' natural pesticides (enzyme inhibitors), proteins or compounds, making them problematic to digest. This in turn causes that low-level inflammation — hard to detect, but a potential setback for our health.

Then don't get me started on stress. Stress can severely interfere with your hormones and affect your cravings. When stressed and/or sleep deprived, we crave sugary foods and drinks which feeds a negative cycle within the gut, causing inflammation.

There are other sources of stress within the body, and we can discuss those later, but for now we can see that poor diet choices can lead to disruption to the gut microbiome. This disruption causes stress and inflammation, ultimately affecting your physical and mental health.

Sugar is also a major contributor to inflammation. This keto diet promotes a low-sugar/low-carb approach in a bid to reduce inflammation and stress on the endocrine system. To adhere to a low-sugar/low-carb diet, it is important to understand the implications of eating a high-sugar/high-carb diet. Note that when I talk about sugar I don't just mean lollies and chocolate bars; I'm also including refined carbohydrates such as pasta, bread, pastries, cakes, pies, croissants . . . you get the picture.

As a response to the carbohydrate (glucose) content in these foods, our pancreas secretes insulin. Insulin then transports glucose to the cell. In normal circumstances the cell is receptive to the delivery of glucose and facilitates its transfer across the cell membrane. The glucose is then used by the cell for energy production.

However, in the current Western eating climate, circumstances are not always normal . . .

Chapter Three

The price of sugar

For years we've been fed the following rhetoric: being underweight or overweight is an energy balance and equates to calories in versus calories out. The model suggests that it's a simple case of adjusting your calorie intake or manipulating your energy expenditure to manage your weight. This isn't necessarily wrong, but there is more to this picture than just calories.

It actually depends on where you are getting those calories from . . . and knowing this is the game changer. If the majority of those calories are derived from carbohydrates, you'll be stimulating the insulin response, and over time this can be problematic.

INSULIN

As previously mentioned, insulin is the vehicle that transports glucose from the bloodstream to the cell. There are sites on the cell membrane that recognise insulin and welcome it with open arms. Think of it as like seeing an old friend at your front door for the first time in ages . . . you'd swing that door open and usher him or her right in. When this happens again and again, the sites become less enthusiastic about insulin, as you would about seeing your old friend if they turned up at your front door several times a day. Over time your cells become desensitised to insulin, and instead of glucose being transported into the cells for energy, the glucose has no choice but to remain in circulation. Consequently, as a direct result of elevated blood glucose, a signal is sent to the pancreas to release more insulin. This doesn't fix the problem; it only serves to have raised insulin.

Ultimately this scenario is highly confusing for your body — your cells aren't receiving the energy and the subsequent signals that tell your body you're satiated — and this leads to higher consumption of foods . . . and we know how this ends.

Without dietary intervention or macronutrient manipulation, your cells can become not only desensitised to insulin but downright resistant to it — otherwise known as type 2 diabetes.

ELEVATED INSULIN

Just like your overzealous friend knocking on your door several times a day, there comes a point in time when you stop answering the door and they bugger off to walk the streets. When this happens to insulin and it has nowhere to go, it sends a signal to denote that food must be in abundance. Pretty simple, really: raised blood glucose means raised insulin levels, which suggests that food must be in abundance — *a reminder that we are simply hunter–gatherers with mobile phones!*

The body's MO is always survival, so in this scenario the elevated insulin signals a need to store fat in preparation for leaner times. We are naturally engineered to gorge on carbohydrates as a mechanism for survival — our ancestors would have only accessed carbs at certain times of the year and gone nuts for it, knowing that leaner months were around the corner. But in today's society winter never comes; food is always in abundance.

Insulin resistance equates to eating nothing, because the cells aren't receiving the energy so the signals aren't being made to let the body know you're full and to stop eating. At this point you're eating empty calories, effectively.

So the take-home message is, calories in versus calories out as a determining factor for weight management lacks substance. We need to dig a little deeper and acknowledge where those calories are coming from, because there is an extra 'cost' when calories are coming from carbohydrates.

DIABETES

There are almost 3.7 million people diagnosed with diabetes in the UK. That's a truckload of people! Add to that the number of people who are experiencing insulin desensitivity (pre-diabetes) but have not yet been diagnosed and the situation becomes alarming.

Type 1 diabetes is an auto-immune disease — the body's immune system attacks the cells in the pancreas that produce insulin, which regulates the blood's glucose levels. If you have type 1 diabetes, you are unable to produce insulin and need daily injections to survive. Type 1 diabetes can occur at any age, although mainly in people under 30 years old.

Type 2 diabetes can be caused by hereditary factors and/or lifestyle, including poor nutrition, lack of exercise and being overweight. If you have type 2 diabetes, you may be able to control it through dietary and other lifestyle changes, but you may also need medication or insulin injections to maintain your blood glucose levels. While type 2 diabetes occurs mainly in people over 40, it is also becoming increasingly common in younger people.

Years ago I was horrified to hear that one of the most successful Olympians of all time, British rower Steve Redgrave (who won gold medals at five consecutive games from 1984 to 2000), was diagnosed with type 2 diabetes. How could Steve Redgrave get diabetes . . . he's so fit and healthy . . . it just doesn't make sense!

To replenish his energy stores from calories exerted during training, Steve had to consume up to 8000 calories a day. The bulk of these calories came from carbohydrates. In order to consume 8000 calories he would have had to been eating A LOT and OFTEN! His insulin then quickly became the overzealous, uninvited, annoying friend at the front door.

Elite athlete or not . . . stressing the metabolic system again and again becomes harmful and will lead to desensitivity to insulin, insulin resistance, elevated blood glucose and insulin, and ultimately fat storage. Diabetes is a hormonal disease and not one driven by an individual's lack of willpower.

OBESITY

Diabetes goes hand in hand with obesity . . . A reliance on carbohydrates feeds this hormonal-disruption scenario, resulting in promotion of fat storage and hunger. As I keep stressing it's not *you*, it's your hormones. Also, for the past 60-odd years we've been led to believe that fat was the bad guy and have eaten carbs with gusto. So it's little wonder we see the incidence of diabetes and obesity we do today.

According to Diabetes UK, three in five women and two in three men are overweight or obese. More than one in three children are overweight or obese by the time they leave primary school in England.

Obesity and diabetes are precursors for many other health implications, BUT the good news is it's all totally reversible.

These conditions are the result of diet choices, and certainly not because of character flaws. By manipulating macronutrients (carbs/fats/protein) it's comforting to know that weight can normalise as well as dramatically reduce systemic inflammation. I've rattled on about real food, inflammation, sugar, diabetes, gut health and obesity – all very necessary to discuss in order to understand the causes, but it's solutions I'm interested in . . . and arguably why you parted with your hard-earned money for this book.

BRAIN HEALTH

I've discussed the implication of sugar on hormones and fat accumulation but it has other ramifications . . . let's explore. If I was to suggest that sugar (carbs) could impact your brain health, you'd probably roll your eyes and accuse me of taking the sugar thing a little too far. But remember, I'm *only* motivated to help you live as healthy a life as possible and that includes fuelling your body AND brain on the right fuel. I want you to look and feel great in your perennial summer body but also *think* sharp too.

As I've suggested in this chapter, it's our inherited genotype to crave sugar and we all have a 'sweet-tooth' to a lesser or greater extent. It's this mechanism that has allowed us to thrive over the last 2 million years – it's promoted the gorging on sweet berries during late summer/ early autumn in preparation for leaner months. However, we are eating like winter is around the corner but it never comes. Hence most of us in the Western world have an overconsumption of sugar/carbs and an absence of healthy fats. How does this affect our brain health?

We are experiencing an epidemic of obesity and diabetes in the Western world but also dementia, with around 850,000 suffering from some form of dementia in the UK, with the number predicted to rise to 2 million by 2051. The rise in neurological conditions is not an anomaly – its driver is the same as obesity and type 2 diabetes – sugar!

Some researchers believe that increased sugar intake correlates with the increasing rate of dementia – suggesting that cells in your brain can become desensitised to insulin, just like other cells elsewhere in your body. Overexposure to sugar can prevent neurons being fed energy simply because the cell becomes resistant to insulin. To measure your blood glucose, ask your doctor for an A1C test – which will tell you your average blood sugar value – this will reflect your insulin sensitivity. In a bid to reduce inflammation and stave off brain disease, reduce your A1C value.

If the majority of your calories are being consumed in the form of carbs, it's fair to assume that other macronutrients (and micronutrients) are being neglected. The brain loves omega 3 and in particular DHA and EPA — available from fish sources or marine algae — however, these valuable brain fuels may be sub-optimal if there is a preference for carbs.

Gluten

When we are talking about brain health and carbohydrates, it's important to address the protein found in many processed foods — gluten. The popularity and availability of gluten-free foods are certainly on the rise, which is encouraging. However, a gluten-free product is certainly not an outright marker of a health product — you will still need to be mindful of reading the labels.

The gravity of gluten as an inflammatory agent should not be undervalued. Although sufferers of coeliac disease only account for 1–2 per cent of the population, and a further 30 per cent for non-coeliac gluten-sensitive folks, the rest of us might not exhibit any intestinal disturbances when exposed to gluten — however, this should not give us the green light to indulge in gluten-laden carbs as the disturbances could be felt cognitively.

If you are a coeliac or know a coeliac, you'll have an understanding of just how reactive gluten can be for health — upon digesting or contact with gluten, there are tangible/visceral symptoms. When the symptoms are more subversive, as in the case of most of us in society, it makes it harder to make the decision to minimise gluten from the diet, simply because there are no/few tangible benefits.

Remember that the cornerstone to diseases or ill-health is inflammation. Not only can gluten potentially cause inflammation of the gut but it can also have devastating consequences for the brain. We now understand the profound relationship between the disruption to blood sugar and neurological conditions such as Alzheimer's disease or dementia. Having a diet high in carbs can increase inflammation and the risk of neurological conditions.

Elevated blood glucose promotes a process called glycation — this is characterised by an increase in blood glucose (can be mild elevation) and a binding to proteins, resulting in two negatives outcomes:

1. Glycation increases the production of free radicals which are potentially harmful to our cells
2. Glycated proteins (binded to sugar) dramatically increase the process of inflammation

The constant theme throughout this book is inflammation and learning what causes it but importantly what are the tricks and tools to minimising inflammation. Part of this picture is focusing on gluten — gluten is a protein found in many carbs and found in wheat, barley and rye products as well as many processed food products. It is a protein that the human body is not designed to accept. As a consequence it causes inflammation as it evokes an immune response — it's this mechanism that is troublesome. So, again, even if you have no intestinal reaction to gluten, it WILL be causing inflammation which can affect you neurologically.

On the consumption of gluten, the protein can cross-react with other proteins within the gut. Gluten unlocks another protein called zonulin — which will increase the permeability of the gut lining. At this point food particles and proteins cross the gut wall which will challenge the immune system. Essentially gluten stimulates other proteins which compromise the gut integrity — paving the way for inflammation.

What's the take-home message here?

Embracing gluten-free products is only one part of the solution . . . but it's a step in the right direction. Knowing that gluten sparks an immune response leading to inflammation, which can be felt in the digestive tract BUT certainly not limited to, is pivotal to health and longevity. Gluten promotes systemic inflammation, the trigger and cause for a myriad of health complications, neurological disease being one of those. The other part of the solution is to reduce sugar and refined carbs in a bid to mitigate glycation.

It is also important to note that gluten sparks a secondary problem that is more silent and subversive, but no less harmful. The antibodies that attack gluten also attack enzymes with similar characteristics to gluten. These enzymes are called transglutaminase 2, 3 and 6.

Transglutaminase 2 is typically found in the gut, and attacks on it cause damage to gut tissue. Transglutaminase 3 is typically found in the skin, so the antibodies attacking it cause skin conditions such as eczema — 30 per cent of people with coeliac disease also present with skin issues. Transglutaminase 6 is typically found in the brain. When the antibodies attack these enzymes, brain health is compromised. If you want to read further on this subject, have a look at www.ncbi.nlm. nih.gov/pubmed/ and search for 'non-coeliac gluten problems'.

CAVEAT

As I briefly mentioned, gluten-free products are on the rise — our supermarket aisles are awash with them . . . but this is not the gold standard for health. I strongly advise you to scrutinise the nutritional panel — the product could still contain sugar, additives, processed oils . . . so be your own food detective. Your body will love you for it.

While we are on the topic of labels (I'll address this later in the book), brands are quick to market their product in the best possible light — be it 'organic', 'gluten-free', 'sugar-free' or 'hand-pressed by virgin-elves' — but it's all marketing tactics. Put your food detective hat on, and once you learn what to look for it'll take seconds to scan a nutritional panel to determine whether a product is worthy of your basket or not. Please don't put all your trust in manufacturers — it's perfectly acceptable to have some scepticism when browsing the items in a supermarket — remember it's YOUR health and so YOU need to be in the driver's seat.

Okay, so what does a diet look like that minimises the systemic inflammation in our body, doesn't stress the hormone insulin, is kind to your gut and isn't restrictive — plus you won't lose your mind counting calories or weighing your food? *The approach is simply a low-carb/ high-fat diet.*

Let me break it down for you.

Chapter Four

What is ketosis?

Adopting a low-carb/high-fat diet by simply manipulating your macronutrients will have significant implications for your health. We can now accept that the health message of the last 60-odd years (low fat, high carb) simply has not worked in our favour, so it's time to rethink this picture. Since the 1950s we have witnessed improvements in farming, leaps in technology, medical advances and improved diagnostic skills, yet our health continues to decline, with epidemics of diabetes, obesity and Alzheimer's disease being seen across the globe. The elephant in the room has been carbohydrates.

Let's look that elephant straight in the eye.

I've gone over the health implications for eating a high-carb diet, so we don't need to reiterate that. Besides, I want to showcase *healthful* foods and celebrate those. When adopting a low-carb protocol, for optimal health it should be accompanied with a high-fat approach. Pairing low carb with high protein comes with its own set of complications — more on this later.

The ketogenic diet has attracted widespread attention recently, primarily due to its many health benefits. The positive ramifications for adopting a ketogenic diet, even periodically, are vast. Being in ketosis will . . .

Encourage fat loss

In my mind, this is a by-product of the pursuit of health — not the driver. Being in ketosis will naturally increase satiety and help to normalise blood sugar levels, assisting with cravings. To produce ketones, your body will need to 'liberate' body fat for metabolism. It is this process in combination with appetite suppression and reduced insulin that will stimulate fat loss.

Improve cognitive function and mood

Ketosis will up-regulate mitochondrial biogenesis, literally creating more power stations in your brain. Ketones have been shown to be the preferred fuel source for the brain and heart, and are able to cross the blood–brain barrier with ease, making them readily available as a fuel source. Brain fog has been blamed on elevated ammonia levels and depressed GABA (the 'chilled-out' neurotransmitter) and ketones have been shown to increase GABA signalling and the removal of ammonia, helping improve clarity.

Improve insulin sensitivity

Having elevated insulin levels can work against us, as I have discussed in the previous pages. Elevated insulin inhibits lipolysis, or the burning of fat. During periods of elevated insulin, fat-burning is blunted until such time that insulin returns to normal levels. However, if insulin is chronically high due to insulin insensitivity then fat utilisation is compromised and fat loss harder to achieve.

Reduce inflammation

This is the golden ticket for me. My 60-day Keto Protocol is designed to reduce systemic inflammation — adopting a ketogenic diet will inhibit inflammasomes, which are a part of the innate immune response and promote inflammation.

Promote neuron regeneration

We need to shake off the idea that we are born with a finite number of brain cells and beyond maturation they slowly die off, accelerated by poor diet and lifestyle. Humans actually have the ability to grow new brain cells through a process called neurogenesis, which occurs when your brain produces more BDNF (brain-derived neurotrophic factor) – 'fertiliser' for the brain. There are a few mechanisms to stimulate BDNF and being in ketosis is one.

Protect neuron health

Ketones produced as a direct result of carb restriction elicit a protective response for the brain, which is highly significant in the fight against neurodegenerative diseases. As we age we do tend to see a decline in the integrity of our brain cells. Studies have shown that ketones improve cognitive function in sufferers of Alzheimer's, Parkinson's and MS. In fact, beta-hydroxybutyrate (one of the naturally produced ketones) has been shown to reduce neuronal loss in animal models.

High fat and low carb: a quick snapshot of the benefits

Here's what you can achieve on a keto diet:

- reduced inflammation
- reduced cravings
- increased satiety
- immediate source of energy
- less oxidative stress

- normalised blood sugar levels
- increased insulin sensitivity
- neuron biogenesis
- mitochondrial biogenesis
- decreased cancer risk
- improved mood
- improved cognitive function
- fat loss

KETOSIS

The fundamental benefit of a low-carb diet is to induce a certain metabolic state called ketosis. Ketosis is a state very familiar to humans – one we have experienced for long periods of our lives throughout the millennia we have walked on this planet. As hunter–gatherers, our ancestors would have experienced periods of low calorie intake due to scarcity of foods. Also, they would have favoured fatty foods that provided the highest nutritional yield per output (hunting or foraging). They didn't care about being healthy or looking good for summer; it was about survival. Being efficient with their energy was optimal for this. Survival meant having a strong preference for nutrient-dense fatty tissues and organ meat over less nutrient-dense foods such as berries and grasses.

This scenario meant that our ancestors would have been in ketosis much of the time. Only during times when carbohydrates were more abundant would they have been reliant on an alternative fuel source. It is worth noting that some hunter–gatherer tribes would have had a low carbohydrate intake all year round. For example, Inuits living in tundra regions relied predominantly on a high-fat diet, eating fat-rich seals, whales and fish. Our ability to function on a diet high in fat, or to cope with periods of low calorie intake, has been instrumental in our survival as a species.

THE NITTY-GRITTY OF KETOSIS

When you expose your body to periods of low calorie intake (fasting or starvation), or whilst on a low-carbohydrate diet, your body will naturally use fat as its primary fuel source. This, my friends, is called ketosis.

Ketosis has been studied and researched for 100 years and has been used in a clinical setting to treat various health conditions — primarily, epilepsy. In recent years, further research into the therapeutic properties of ketosis has led to a global movement, one that promotes high fat in the name of health. Such are the advances into the study of ketosis that it is now possible to ingest supplementary ketones to help slip into ketosis. However, for the time being I'm referring to *nutritional* ketosis.

In the absence of carbohydrates, your body mobilises and utilises fat for energy. Fat is carried to the liver and is oxidised, producing three ketones:

1. Acetone
2. Acetoacetate
3. Beta-hydroxybutyrate

These ketones are then released from the liver and become available for energy. The body is a truly miraculous thing: it detects raised blood ketone levels and sets about a process called mitochondrial biogenesis, whereby the cells increase the number of mitochondria. Mitochondria are the little powerhouses within cells that are responsible for creating energy by breaking down an organic compound called adenosine triphosphate (ATP). It stands to reason that the more powerhouses within each cell, the greater the available energy for every bodily function. This is a game changer for general health, but also for athletic performance, enabling an athlete to perform more kilometres or more reps/sets.

I'm sure much of this sounds familiar to you. There are a few buzzwords and food trends that have popped up over the past few years: words and trends like Atkins, paleo, primal, low-sugar, sugar-free and low FODMAP. But how does a high-fat/low-carb diet differ to what has been before?

Let me outline a few influential food trends before I tell you about what makes the keto protocol different.

SUGAR-FREE DIET

It's comforting to realise that the diets I'm describing here all sing a similar song — that carbs or sugar is the common denominator and that there is a need to reduce consumption of these. The sugar-free movement is no different. My first criticism is that adopting a sugar-free lifestyle is unattainable in the long term. If . . . and it's a BIG if . . . you were super-disciplined about removing sugar from your diet, I'd have to question how long you could sustain this for. Are we talking about refined sugar, fruit, artificial sugars, sugar alcohol — what's in and what's out? From my experience over the years, sugar-free adopters simply replace refined (table sugar) with more natural forms of sugar such as honey or maple syrup. A natural sweetener, such as honey, will have a similar physiological impact as table sugar.

Having said that, the sugar-free movement has certainly helped put sugar under the microscope. It has helped encourage people to read food labels and that is a great thing. If this dietary approach is not attainable long term, it certainly acts like a sugar-cleanse and helps people re-evaluate their daily sugar intake. From what I can tell, there is little said on other macronutrients on the diet — if you remove calories through eliminating sugar . . . are we replacing them with anything?

LOW FODMAP

FODMAP is an acronym that stands for 'fermentable oligosaccharides, disaccharides, monosaccharides and polyols'. It's been identified that if these compounds are poorly absorbed they'll consequently ferment in the large intestine and cause irritable bowel syndrome (IBS). Reducing foods that contain FODMAPs, including onion, garlic, artichoke, honey, pear, leek, milk, barley, wheat and rye, can help to alleviate IBS symptoms.

The low FODMAP approach is essentially an elimination diet — whereby all potential suspects are removed for a period of time, then selectively reintroduced. I like this approach to health in that you treat your own body as a case study, find a path back to health, and then further optimise your health. The low FODMAP diet sets about relieving symptoms of IBS which can be crippling for sufferers. Many of us reassess our lifestyle and diet as a consequence of a health condition or scare — my response to this is to simply avoid that scenario prior to it happening.

Be proactive rather than reactive in relation to your health.

THE ATKINS DIET

Dr Robert Atkins was a pioneer for his time. Back in the 1970s he suggested that it was the high-carbohydrate diet that was the root cause of poor health in the Western world. He introduced the term ketosis to the American public, but due to it sounding incredibly similar to a life-threatening condition for type 1 diabetics called ketoacidosis (extremely high blood glucose plus elevated ketones), he circled back around that and focused on a low-carb diet rather than a high-fat diet.

Atkins was very nearly on the money from a nutritional point of view. However, to my mind there were some flaws in his approach. They were:

1. **A heavy focus on weight loss.** If we spent more time and energy focusing on health as the goal, I'm convinced it would foster a better paradigm. There is *so* much stress placed upon weight management that failure to achieve the ideal body can create despair. Couple this with body dysmorphia, images in the media and poor self-esteem and it doesn't take a rocket scientist to realise that it's a minefield when the focus is on weight loss.

2. **Protein happy.** Atkins's low-carb diet gave the green light to protein, and Americans simply threw more turkey in the oven and another hanger steak on the barbecue to compensate for the calories lost in carbs. Here's the low-down on excessive protein: when our body's requirement for protein has been exceeded, protein is converted to glucose and stored as fat. Not only does this stress the insulin response, it also promotes fat storage. Unless you're training heavily or reproducing, 1 gram of protein per kilogram of lean body weight is sufficient.

3. **Lack of integrity around food sovereignty.** Widespread disregard as to where food came from started in the 1970s, and admittedly we haven't improved a great deal since then, but this is worth exploring further. The quality of the food consumed was not a high priority for Atkins's followers, who consumed feedlot cattle and processed oils with little consideration of ethics, nor of the health benefits of eating organic/biodynamic, hormone-free, free-range or pasture-fed proteins.

THE PALEO DIET

First brought to the public domain by Dr Loren Cordain in 1999, this diet encouraged us to eat like our ancestors of more than 10,000 years ago. It advocated avoiding grains, dairy products and legumes, and celebrating foods such as fish, game, poultry, nuts, seeds and offal. Attention was given to avoiding highly processed foods — essentially building upon the Atkins diet of the 1970s.

On a great many levels the paleo diet works for health, but this only really applies when you pursue a purist paleo diet – one that is marked by high fat, low carb and the elimination of certain food groups.

The mass uptake of the diet led to reinterpretations that weren't always positive. These included:

1. **Overconsumption of protein.** Similar to the Atkins diet, followers ate protein with gusto. Rather than making up the lost calories from carbs with fat, followers plugged the hole with protein.

2. **Uncertain food quality.** Again, like the Atkins diet, little attention was placed on food traceability. Not noting or caring where the food comes from exposed a set of health problems.

3. **Bacon, bacon, bacon . . .** Google search 'paleo meals' online and if it's not served with bacon, I'll eat my Akubra. I'm confident the pork industry loved the spike in bacon sales, but putting it simply, there are better meat choices than bacon (*unless* you are mindful of where it comes from and what's been added to it).

4. **You say potato, I say sweet potato . . .** With little reference to macronutrients with the modern paleo diet, carbs in the form of sweet potato slipped through the net. Seen as a powerhouse of nutrients, the sweet potato was hailed as the king of veggies. However, the net carb value of sweet potato is fairly high (1 cup = 22.76 grams, whereas 1 cup of broccoli is 3.64 grams). So although a *real food*, the sweet potato feeds the hormonal cycle of blood glucose and insulin. The bottom line is, sweet potato is a glycaemic food – one that spikes blood sugar.

5. **Paleo treats. Oh, don't get me started!** One of the biggest merits of the paleo diet was its aversion to processed foods and ingredients, and that it encouraged folks to read labels. This naturally meant that treats such as M&Ms were on the banned substances list. But while M&Ms sat on the shelves getting dusty, it opened the door for the wolf in sheep's clothing: the paleo treat. Suddenly, treats were being made sweetened with wholefoods and natural foods

such as dates, prunes, honey, agave and maple syrup. However, the bottom line is that sugar is sugar is sugar: it will elicit the same physiological response whatever its source.

'PRIMAL DIET'

The 'primal diet' was borne out of the paleo diet. Where they diverge is paleo practitioners have strong views on legumes and dairy, but the primal diet approach is slightly less dogmatic. The primal approach acknowledges that *some* types of dairy can be healthful. Dairy that is fermented, raw and from grass-fed animals is acceptable. The diet also acknowledges that legumes are a source of prebiotics.

Primal is more than just a diet, it incorporates a lifestyle — including movement, and a tolerance to the occasional 'treat' if that makes you content. It embraces coffee, which is a big plus for me. My 60-day Keto Protocol has more crossover with the primal diet than the paleo diet in that it is a lifestyle rather than a diet that restricts. Comparing primal and paleo isn't like comparing apples and oranges — there are only mild differences, with primal being a little less dogmatic — which may be the reason behind its success. Folks who have explored or trialled the primal diet will see similarities with my 60-day protocol.

•

In order to evolve towards the optimal diet for humans, it's necessary to embrace the positives of trends gone by and disregard or sideline the negatives. There's an element of trial and error, in combination with current research. These two factors will facilitate the 'natural order of things'.

What do I mean by that?

With enough people investing in health from a clinical perspective, as well as 'everyday folk' trialling foods and supplements in order to optimise their health, soon enough the right information will naturally rise to the top. At this point, most of the hard work has been done for us and we can cherry-pick the most current, robust information to help us on the path to optimal health. I'm not suggesting that all roads lead to a single diet that suits every single person on this planet — that will never happen — but there is certainly great information out there which will benefit us all from a health perspective.

UNPACKING KETOSIS

Getting into ketosis really isn't that hard — most of us experience it at many points in our lives. Some of us will regularly wake up in ketosis. Any time you have been calorie restricted through illness, fasting or manipulating your carbs, you will have been in ketosis.

Measuring whether you're in or out of ketosis isn't hard. Being in ketosis is defined as having elevated blood ketone levels, generally regarded between 0.5–3 millimoles. There are a number of ways to monitor ketone levels: blood, breath or urine tests. All methods have pros and cons, from accuracy to affordability, but generally speaking blood monitors are considered the most accurate. They measure the level of beta-hydroxybutyrate in the blood. Blood ketone monitors can be bought online or in some pharmacies.

It might seem quite extreme to be measuring your blood, but if you're a new adopter of this dietary approach, you might welcome having tangible evidence as to whether or not you are in ketosis. Once you get used to how it feels to be in this state, you probably won't need to check, you will just know.

So let's suggest you ate dinner early, and that dinner consisted of a low-carb meal. You then went to bed, and when you woke up you had to skip breakfast and rush out the door. By lunchtime (if not upon waking) you'd most likely be in ketosis. At this point you begin to reap the therapeutic properties of being in ketosis.

This is a doddle, right?!

Unaccustomed (at this point) to a high-fat diet or to fasting, you begin to get hunger signals, leading to cravings, so you reach out for a snack. It could be a sushi roll, a banana, some dried fruit or a ham sandwich. At this point the dumping of glucose (rice, fruit sugar and grain respectively) into your system is enough to knock you out of ketosis, and you once again become a carbohydrate-burning machine. This illustrates the ease in which we can get into ketosis, but also the ease in which we can get knocked out. It's not critical to stay in ketosis 100 per cent of the time, plus it's unrealistic. Staying in ketosis at least *most* of the time will be easier once you become fat-adapted.

'Fat-adapted' is a term used to describe the up-regulation of various pathways to ensure you can utilise and metabolise fat efficiently. This fat adaptation doesn't happen overnight; rather, it takes several weeks for the up-regulation of fat-burning enzymes and mitochondrial biogenesis to take place . . . but rest assured it will happen.

FASTING

As I've mentioned there are a number of pathways to get to nutritional ketosis, and fasting is one of them. Fasting has been used throughout the ages and is an integral part of various religions. Whatever your motivation for fasting, the outcome is pretty much the same — you'll switch your fuel source from carbs to fat. If you have never deliberately fasted before and are currently on a high-carb diet, it will most likely feel uncomfortable and the hunger signals will be strong; however, when you fast when fat-adapted, it won't feel quite as hellish . . . in fact, it's fairly effortless.

There are two ways to think about fasting: fasting for cognitive function, and fasting for cellular health.

Whether or not you're in nutritional ketosis prior to a fast, the very act of fasting will most likely force you into ketosis anyway. As we know, elevated blood ketones is achieved through carbohydrate restriction *or* starvation. Going without food will promote the natural production of ketones, which are then released into the circulatory system and used by cells, your heart and your brain. Unlike fat, which is hydrophobic, the ketones are able to cross the blood–brain barrier and become available for fuel for the brain. You've probably heard, over the years, that your brain needs glucose (carbs) to survive. This isn't necessarily false, but our liver can produce the required glucose in isolation of dietary carbs, so there's no need to eat bagels for your brain to keep ticking over.

Anecdotal evidence of improved cognitive function and alertness experienced while fasting is compelling. The fact that the ketogenic diet up-regulates mitochondrial biogenesis in the brain suggests that more energy can be supplied to the brain.

From my experience of being in ketosis, either through fasting, adjusting my macronutrients or via exogenous ketones (supplements), I've noticed increased focus, improved cognitive function and better recall. I'll use this to my advantage, too: if I have an important meeting, a presentation to give or just need to be 'on', I'll engineer it so I'm reaping the benefits of being in ketosis at the same time. I've even taken exogenous ketones an hour before going on a date. (The fact that I remain single is not reflective of the ketones, I'm sure!)

When the body experiences a period of starvation, it triggers a certain energetic pathway to promote 'cleansing' . . . from a cellular level. I examine this process a little more deeply in the next chapter but for now, consider that our bodies have two energetic pathways.

The first one is an anabolic pathway and responsible for cellular growth and cell division – think anabolic steroids . . . things get bigger!

This is a necessary pathway, and a familiar one if you're training. It is called mTOR.

The second pathway is responsible for cell rejuvenation, so rather than the cell responding to stress to divide and grow, it removes dead cell components, toxins and cleanses. This is called cell autophagy.

The relationship between one pathway and another means that when one is activated the opposing is stifled. Therefore, whilst mTOR is activated the cleansing of a cell won't occur. If this scenario is left unchecked, the unwanted dead cell components and toxins can be detrimental to your health. It's completely normal and optimal to swing from one pathway to another, but having autophagy inhibited for long periods is unhealthy.

Therefore, it's wise to periodically cleanse your cells, allowing for the removal of damaged cell components, dead cell components and toxins. This cleansing process is seen in the brain, too, with fasting promoting neuronal autophagy (self-eating). Without it, the brain does not grow or function as it should.

The bottom line about fasting is that it is a potent, not to mention cheap, method to greatly affect the health of our cells and mitochondria.

There are many perspectives on frequency and duration of fasts. My recommendations would be:

1. Aim for 16+ hours.
2. Start with once a month, progressing to once a fortnight and ultimately once or twice a week.
3. Every quarter, try a longer fast — 2–3 days.
4. Increase the length of your fasts as you become more comfortable with them and more fat-adapted.
5. Have an early dinner the night before (sleep is counted as fasting time).
6. Drink plenty of water.

7. Break the fast with a fat-rich meal/snack to help the body to become fat-adapted.
8. Buddy up. Having support will be beneficial in the initial instance.

Fasting is just one tool to amplify health, and when worked in together with good nutrition, exercise, rest, recovery and smart supplementation will dramatically influence your epigenetics, turning on life-enhancing genes.

For now, however, your task is to achieve ketosis through restricting carbs and amplifying fats. On the following page is my ketosis story, to give you an idea of what might be in store for you.

Epigenetics

Here's a brief explanation of why this topic gets me excited. If you've never come across the word 'epigenetics', it simply means *gene expression can be influenced by age, lifestyle and diet*. To think that we can alter the direction of our longevity, health and happiness through external factors is perhaps nothing new, but knowing that this happens on a cellular level makes it very tangible.

We know that food is information and will directly influence our hormones and ultimately our gene expression – the bottom line is that we are not set in stone. Wherever you may be on the health spectrum and whatever age you are, it's possible to influence your health positively through turning health-promoting genes 'on' through diet and lifestyle.

According to nutritional sciences researcher Associate Professor Dominic D'Agostino, beta-hydroxybutyrate (one of the ketones our liver produces) functions to 'turn on' genes that are neuro-protective and cellular-protective – which are linked to longevity pathways. Simply knowing this, to me, is a potent reminder that we can control so many facets of our health, from gut health, to cognitive function and immunity. Every mealtime is an opportunity to nourish our body with healthful 'information'. Every meal, snack and drink can contribute to the overall, bigger picture of health.

I'm not implying you're a ticking time-bomb and the wrong foods at lunch will trigger a cascading effect – this scare-tactic will only lead to unhealthy behaviours around food. Food needs to be enjoyed, so being informed will help you to still enjoy food whilst simultaneously promoting optimal health.

I guess I'm hoping you get as excited as I do about epigenetics – it's a fascinating area of discussion. Food . . . is information. Food . . . is more than simply a calorie. Food . . . is instruction for genetic expression. Food . . . is interacting with our genome. Food . . . is more than macro- and micronutrients. Food . . . can amplify health and longevity.

FROM THE HORSE'S MOUTH – MY KETOSIS STORY

Whilst I've been trying to eat clean for a while now, it was four or five years ago that I started dabbling with a really high fat diet . . . and manipulating my macronutrients accordingly. At the time I was entrenched in the paleo diet and knee-deep in sweet potato, which is high in carbs and would certainly have been preventing me from being in ketosis. So I took steps to ensure I would be in nutritional ketosis, getting up to 80–85 per cent of my calories from fat, 10–15 per cent from protein and the rest from carbs. To be honest, it wasn't much of a challenge with paleo being my starting point, for as I've mentioned before, a *purist paleo* diet is close to a ketogenic diet.

At that time it was my habit to train six days a week, predominantly doing plyometrics ('explosive movement') and high-intensity stuff. I was in my late 30s and had been training all my life. Therefore, if there were going to be any changes to my output as a direct result of my diet, I reasoned that I'd notice it, however subtle the change.

Well, let me tell you, there was nothing subtle about it! Training now felt like hell — like training in wet cement whilst wearing oversized wellies. High-intensity training is never a walk in the park, but because my body was now relying on a different fuel, things were different. It was like I didn't have the 'infrastructure' to deal with the energy demand on that fuel. But I knew from my reading that the human body is able to quickly adapt to ensure energy demand is met. All that needed to happen was an up-regulation of mitochondria (the cells' power stations) and up-regulation of fat-burning enzymes and I'd be sweet.

I don't recall exactly how long it took, but after a few weeks I noticed a positive shift in energy, with heightened mood, increased concentration and improved cognitive function. I also noticed a distinct 'constant' with my energy throughout the day. All this I found very alluring. Don't get me wrong, I'm not impervious to tiredness, but I felt that my food was energising me, rather than pinning me to the lounge like a bowl of pasta would.

I was keen to continue experimenting with this high-fat low-carb protocol just to see what happened to my body over time. The biggest observable shift was with training and my output in the gym. I remember one day going in and feeling amazing — kind of invincible. My programme that day wasn't anything out of the ordinary but I smashed it like it was a workout for a toddler. I started to dissect what was different. Had I timed my coffee perfectly on the way to the gym? Had I eaten a nutritionally perfect meal? Was it a full moon? Was my Saturn returning? Before I drove myself nuts with wondering, I decided to see how my performance was the following day.

It was the same: I struggled to feel fatigued. I felt like I had 10–20 per cent more to give within my session.

I acknowledge that my findings are only anecdotal, but the results were compelling enough for me to continue with the diet and do further research. I'd trained all my life and nothing had come close to this as a training/performance aid. I'd dabbled with supplements and a myriad of superfoods over the years, but from a training perspective the reliance on ketones eclipsed everything.

KETO FLU

Let's say tomorrow you want to begin your ketosis journey, after having enjoyed a carb-rich diet for most of your life. As has already been explained, this can be achieved via two methods: fasting and carb restriction.

As your body transitions from carbohydrates as a primary fuel source to fats, expect to feel pretty ordinary. The body is equipped to run on fat *or* carbs. It's also capable of converting protein to carbohydrate for fuel. This versatility has allowed us to survive on this planet for millennia. But just like any mechanism, things may not run all that smoothly first time around, particularly if that mechanism hasn't been used for 10, 20, 30 or 40 years. Until the dust has been blown off and the cogs oiled, the machinery moans and groans. This is called the keto flu.

It was the keto flu that I experienced when I first put myself on a low-carb diet. It took a number of days before I felt any benefits, and even longer until my training resembled anything like normal (remember me in my wellies trudging through wet cement?).

Not all of us will experience the keto flu when transitioning, but if you are one of the unlucky ones, expect some of the following symptoms:

- brain fog
- headaches/migraines

- light-headedness/dizziness
- irritability

It's important not to jump back on the carb train when you experience these symptoms. Faced with adversity, it's human nature to resort to something familiar and comforting, which in this case might be a bowl of pasta or ice-cream. But don't fall for this. Until your machinery is fully operational, expect to feel lousy.

However, there are a number of tricks you can employ to mitigate the symptoms.

1. Increase the consumption of fatty fish or fish oil

Research has shown that, through low-carb diets or rapid weight loss, arachidonic acid is released into the bloodstream from stored adipose tissue (fat). This can cause headaches by increasing inflammatory molecules. Fatty fish like sardines and mackerel can help to buffer the effects of the inflammatory molecules.

2. Increase your salt intake

In a nutshell, for each gram of carbohydrate stored in the body there's around 2–2.4 grams of water. When carbohydrate intake is restricted then its stored version (glycogen) is depleted too. With that comes a reduction in water. This is often the reason people experience initial rapid weight-loss when cutting out carbs. However, the water contains many minerals, including sodium, so it's necessary to increase your salt intake. Restricting carbs will usually mean eating fewer refined foods, which are often riddled with sodium, therefore don't be shy of seasoning your foods with some good sea salt to redress the balance.

3. Increase potassium

Similar to sodium, potassium is lost as a direct result of a reduction of water in the body. Ensure this electrolyte is replaced through real foods such as avocados and leafy greens.

4. Increase magnesium

Magnesium is another electrolyte lost, so be sure to redress the balance with magnesium-rich foods (spinach, chard and pumpkin seeds), or consider a supplement.

5. Drink more water

By now you're hopefully beginning to see that loss of water has a big impact. On a carb-restricted diet you'll need to consume more water. A rule of thumb is to multiple your body weight by 0.04 to get daily consumption in litres. For me it's 85 kg × 0.04 = 3.4 litres. Another rule of thumb is to ensure you have two clear pees in the middle of the day.

6. Include some MCT oil

MCT will pop up a number of times in this book. It stands for medium-chain triglycerides, which are converted in the liver to ketones to be a readily available source of energy. Coconut oil is an example of a food which is high in MCT, but pure MCT oil is what you're after. It's been around for decades and can be found in most health-food stores or supermarkets. Look for C8 and C10 — this is caprylic acid and capric acid respectively, which is the gold you're after. Essentially, consuming MCT will help you propagate your own ketones and help with the low-carb transitioning process. I've been taking MCT for years and have it daily in my coffee (see recipe page 253), in my smoothie or straight off a spoon.

A warning: MCT is clear and devoid of taste, making it easy to consume; however, it can cause some gastric disturbances. Within 10–20 minutes of ingesting it, it *can* give you a stomach ache (of around five minutes' duration), and can induce a bowel movement. So my advice is to start with 1 teaspoon and progress to 3–5 tablespoons over a few weeks.

7. Ketone supplements

Ketone supplements, otherwise known as exogenous ketones (meaning outside the body, as opposed to endogenous: inside), effectively flood your body with beta-hydroxybutyrate. Being one of the three ketones that we naturally manufacture, beta-hydroxybutyrate increases our blood ketone levels and can certainly help to transition into nutritional ketosis when restricting carbs. I've personally taken exogenous ketones periodically over the last 18 months and can report improved mood as well as improved cognitive function and recall. There are a few ketone supplements on the market. If you can find a product that has a combination of BHB and MCT in its formula, then this is preferential in propagating your own ketones.

8. Gradually reduce carbs

Giving up carbs is no different from giving up any habit that you've had for years – it's hard! Actually, giving up carbs is incredibly difficult, due to the dopamine response that eating carbs elicits. Dopamine is a neurotransmitter that controls the brain's reward/pleasure centre. Long-term exposure to carbs can lead to dependency on them. One solution is to ease into a low-carb diet, reducing daily intake gradually.

THE PROTOCOL: OLD VERSUS NEW KETO DIET

It's important to distinguish the protocol for ketosis. In other words, what macronutrient breakdown do we have to follow in order to become fat-burning machines? The truth is there is no hard and fast rule. There are certain parameters, of course, but 'classic keto' – which was first described in the 1920s when the diet was used to treat kids with epilepsy — has been superseded by a modern version which may be the key to adherence for the broader population.

CLASSIC KETO

Back in the 1920s, physician John Hopkins noticed that when juvenile epileptic patients were calorie restricted, the frequency of the seizures reduced. Upon taking blood samples of the patients, the level of raised ketones was noted, and hence the approach was coined the keto diet.

The classic keto diet works on a ratio of 4:1 or 3:1, which is a little confusing but makes more sense when explained as a percentage of daily calories.

The ratio 4:1 refers to 4 grams of fat to 1 gram of protein/carbs. When translated to a percentage of calories for each macronutrient, it equates to:

Classic keto 4:1	fat	protein	carbohydrate
	92%	7%	1%

The ratio 3:1 refers to 3 grams of fat to 1 gram of protein/carbs. When translated to a percentage of calories for each macronutrient, it equates to:

Classic keto 3:1	fat	protein	carbohydrate
	88%	9%	3%

The limitation with classic keto is that it's often hard to consume 90 per cent of your daily calories through fat. Fat is arguably less palatable than carbs or protein. A problem that can potentially stem from this protocol is that followers don't consume enough total calories and risk becoming malnourished. There is also a risk of not taking in adequate amounts of protein, which comes with its own set of problems.

Classic keto is tricky to adhere to. It will work in a clinical environment, where patients are hospitalised and macronutrients are weighed and measured, but for individuals trying it at home, it is a challenge.

MODIFIED KETO OR MODIFIED ATKINS DIET

Recognising that the classic keto diet might be hard to stick to for Joe Bloggs, a compromise has been found which still facilitates ketosis and has all the therapeutic benefits associated with it, but which is a little more practical.

The calorie intake for a modified keto diet looks like:

	fat	*protein*	*carbohydrate*
Modified keto	75%	15–20%	5–10%

The 10 per cent intake of carbs is from non-glycaemic (non-starchy) carbs. Carbs in this category include Brussels sprouts, broccoli, cabbage, spinach, kale, asparagus and mushrooms.

If you're beginning to wonder where all your fat-derived calories are going to come from, here's a snapshot list of some staples:

salmon	duck fat	walnuts
mackerel	MCT oil	pecans
sardine	liver	olive oil
anchovies	kidney	avocado
coconut oil	bone marrow	olives
butter	coconut cream	eggs
beef dripping	coconut milk	cacao
ghee	coconut butter	cocoa butter
lard	macadamias	tahini

Some of the foods on this list might be alien to you now. However, once in the swing of a higher-fat diet, it'll all become second nature. Plus the exciting thing is that fat carries lots of flavour, so your creations will be oozing with deliciousness.

From now on when I'm referring to a high-fat diet I'm referring to the *modified* keto diet, the one that represents 75 per cent calories from fat.

Okay, so let's get started and explore some of the strategies for success.

Chapter Five

Staying on track

Switching from a predominately carbohydrate diet to a high-fat diet can be confronting and confusing, and there's a risk you'll fall off the wagon before it leaves the station, so here are a few strategies that might help.

BUDDY UP

'A problem shared is a problem halved . . .' I'm not sure if that's the most appropriate adage, but you catch my drift. Perhaps 'safety in numbers' is a little better? Anyway, having a buddy to bounce ideas off, share recipes with, eat alongside and provide a sounding board with how you're feeling will be invaluable. It will help if your buddy is a member of your household or someone you work with (as opposed to a Facebook friend living in Kyrgyzstan . . . though I'm not discounting social media as a legit platform for support). Let's face it, the more dialogue you have with a person or people, the better.

DEXA SCAN

By no means is this a prerequisite of starting out, but it will provide an interesting baseline to work from. A DEXA scan (an advanced form of X-ray technology) is a full body-composition scan which will provide you with accurate results relating to your body composition. It will detail your fat mass, lean tissue, bone density, level of hydration, and much more. I get a DEXA scan done periodically, more out of curiosity than anything, to track whether eating and training protocols have affected my body composition.

BLOOD TEST

Again, like the DEXA scan, this is certainly not essential or a prerequisite, but it will give you a reference point. Ask your GP for a full blood panel. Aim to retest 12 weeks into the high-fat diet.

Store-cupboard

Simply having temptation foods in the house might be enough to steer you off course. The best way to avoid this is to spring-clean your store-cupboard and fridge.

OUT

vegetable oil	confectionery
rapeseed oil	pasta
safflower oil	rice
sunflower oil	ice-cream
margarine	fruit roll-ups
biscuits	bread
cakes	table salt
cocoa (heated cacao)	

REMOVE TEMPTATION

You don't have to be a rocket scientist to know that if treats are not in the house then it's hard to consume them. I know we live in an age of delivery eats, but try to avoid these services. Removing temptation will be critical to adherence and success, particularly in the early stages of transitioning to high fat/low carb. I'm not suggesting that everything containing carbs is on the banned substances list, but in a bid to forge new behaviours around food it might be wise to remove all temptations for the time being — just until your cravings have subsided and fat adaptation has taken place.

READ THE LABEL

If you don't currently read labels then I strongly suggest you start. Knowing what's in the food you are ingesting can be critical for general health. Have you ever noticed that a bunch of kale doesn't contain a label? That's because it is what it is! The further something is from its natural source, or that is engineered in a laboratory, the more ingredients it will have.

Most processed foods come with long lists of ingredients. From both a keto and a health perspective, it's vital to know what is in ingredients. Is it carb-heavy, does it contain lots of sugars, fillers, additives? These are all important things to cross-check. The ingredients at the top of the list constitute the primary ingredients, as you move down the list the ingredients become lesser in overall volume. However, the volume (percentage of total volume) of a particular ingredient will not denote how harmful or inflammatory it is. For instance, an ingredient near the bottom of the list with low volume can still have adverse effects. Over time you'll learn what to look for. When scanning labels, look for MORE than just macros such as carbs and sugars — dissect it with a fine-tooth comb for weird and wonderful ingredients.

Here's a rule of thumb: if there are more than five or six ingredients, and/or you struggle to pronounce some of those ingredients, give the product a wide berth.

Reading carbs

Nutritional panels will show Total Carbohydrate. This is important, but it's also important to factor in the net carbs. This will be critical to you staying in ketosis. Net carbs are total carbs minus fibre. Although fibre is technically a carb, the configuration of molecules means they don't enter your bloodstream, therefore won't impact blood glucose/insulin. To achieve ketosis, aim for around 30—40 g net carbs per day.

Sugar in its many guises

Manufacturers have devised clever strategies to circumvent the labelling of 'sugar' on their products. Instead of declaring xx grams of sugar, they use other forms of sugar, most of which are unknown to the masses, thus pulling the wool over our eyes. Below is a list of the types of sugars manufacturers use, some of which I'm sure will be instantly recognisable to you, but others of which I'm equally sure are foreign to you. Etch these names in your subconscious: agave, blackstrap molasses, brown sugar, cane crystal, barley malt, beet sugar, brown rice syrup, buttered sugar, cane juice, caramel, carob syrup, caster sugar, coconut sugar, corn sweetener, corn syrup, crystalline fructose, date sugar, demerara sugar, dextran, diastic malt powder, diastase, ethyl maltol, evaporated cane juice, fructose, galactose, glucose, golden sugar . . .

This is tiring . . . haha

. . . golden syrup, high fructose corn syrup, honey, invert sugar, lactose, malt syrup, maltodextrin, maltose, maple syrup, molasses syrup, muscovado sugar, raw sugar, oat syrup, panela, panocha, rice bran syrup, sorghum syrup, sucrose, treacle, tapioca syrup, turbinado sugar, yellow sugar . . . to name but a few!

While we are on the subject of sugar and labels, measurements are always expressed as grams, which can mean very little. But keep in the back of your mind that 4 grams = 1 teaspoon and you'll be on your way to deciphering sugar amounts.

Serving sizes

When you're reading labels, in addition to examining the nutrition panel it's worth taking a look at the serving size. Manufacturers can be sneaky at times and give you nutritionals based on an unrealistic serving size. The serving size for ice-cream, for example, might be ½ cup, but cast your eyes on a ½ cup measure and consider whether that constitutes an average serve for most of us. We might *start* with a ½-cup serve but then go back for a second and third . . . Bear this in mind particularly when reading labels for breakfast cereals, yoghurts and juices — it's the manufacturers' way of misleading us.

TAKE YOUR OWN LUNCH TO WORK

For me, this ticks a couple of boxes. Ninety-nine per cent of leftovers taste better the next day than they did the day they were cooked, *FACT*. This is particularly the case for curries and slow-cooked dishes . . . and this book is full of mouth-watering recipes for such dishes. Taking your own lunch will ensure you're getting the optimal macronutrients — driving ketosis but eliminating the risk of heading out for a 'convenient' lunch. We all know that healthy lunch options can be limited. Things are improving, but by and large most offerings come in the form of sandwiches, pasta and other carbs. It's these ingredients that carry a glycaemic load and will knock you out of ketosis — not the end of the world, but long-term we want to minimise the intensity and frequency of the glycaemic load and subsequent hormonal response.

There are a few approaches to making leftovers. Either make a larger-than-normal batch of dinner the night before and throw it in the fridge, or if you're organised and have some time up your sleeve, plan to do a big cook-up on the weekend in order to supply you with enough meals to see you through the week. It's worth noting that there is no magic bullet to achieving health — it *does* require planning, diligence and discipline — but the pay-off is second to none.

BIG COOK-UP

As I mentioned, a big cook-up does require some planning, but having the right attitude will help drive success. Rather than seeing a cook-up as an arduous task, view it as freeing-up time later in the week.

It's possible to streamline your grocery shopping and cooking time by utilising a 'hero' ingredient and then cooking it three ways. Here's an example, using chicken as the central ingredient.

Hero chicken – shopping list

4 brown onions
1 small red onion
2 whole chickens
3 garlic cloves
1 large (approx. 400 g) sweet potato
4 eggs
2 tomatoes
3 ripe avocados
8 baby radicchio leaves
8 baby cos leaves
2–3 celery sticks
2–3 carrots
half a pumpkin or whole butter nut squash
handful of peas (can be frozen)
half a lemon
1–2 limes
1 sprig of lemon thyme
¼ bunch of parsley
¼ bunch of coriander
2 sprigs of thyme
1 bay leaf
¼ cup coconut flour
2 litres chicken broth
2–4 tablespoons butter
1–2 tablespoons coconut oil
6 tablespoons olive oil
sea salt
black pepper
1 teaspoon cumin

1. Preheat your oven to 250°C.

2. *Prepare the chickens* – Peel and halve 2 brown onions. Insert these and half a sprig of lemon thyme into the cavity of each chicken. Make a small incision beneath the skin and breast, insert 1 tablespoon butter and massage in. Place both chickens in a large roasting pun, drizzle each with 2 tablespoons olive oil, and season with salt and pepper. Reduce the oven to 190°C and bake on the highest shelf for 1 hour.

3. *Prepare the onions and garlic* – Peel and finely dice the onions (2 small brown – 1 for fritters, 1 for soup; 1 small red – for tacos) and garlic (3 cloves for soup).

4. *Prepare sweet potato fritters* – Coarsely grate the sweet potato, mix with 4 lightly whisked eggs, 1 of the finely diced brown onions and salt and pepper. You can add a bit of coconut flour at this point if it looks like it needs it to bind. Cover and pop in the fridge until you're ready to cook the fritters.

5. *Prepare the soup* – Chop the carrots and celery. Place a saucepan over medium heat, add 2 tablespoons olive oil, then add all the garlic, 1 of the diced brown onions, the celery, carrot and herbs (1 bay leaf, 2 sprigs of thyme). Stir occasionally for 5–6 minutes, or until the onions have softened. Add 2 litres chicken broth and bring to the boil. Reduce the heat and simmer for 15 minutes.

6. *Prepare the guacamole for the tacos* – Soak the chopped red onion in a bowl of water for 5–10 minutes, rinse and drain. Set aside. Peel and scoop the flesh from 3 avocados into a bowl and mash with a fork. Mix in the red onion, the juice from 1–2 limes, some chopped coriander leaves, and cumin. Place in an airtight container in the fridge.

7. *Start cooking sweet potato fritters* – Place a frying pan over medium heat, add a dollop of butter or coconut oil, then take ¼ of the

sweet potato batter you've already prepared, drop it into the pan and flatten down with the back of a spatula. Cook for 4 minutes on one side, then flip and cook for a further 2 minutes on the other (use a plate on top of the pan to assist with the flipping). Make a further three fritters in the same manner (18 minutes).

8. *Add pumpkin or squash to the soup* – Chop the pumpkin into 2 cm chunks. Put into the saucepan with the rest of the soup ingredients and cook for 15 minutes. Transfer the soup into a blender in batches, blending the mixture for 20 seconds.

9. *Finish the chickens* – Remove the chickens from the oven and allow to rest for 10 minutes. Season the chicken meat from one of the chickens and serve with the fritters for dinner tonight (Night 1).

10. *Finish the soup* – Put the blended soup back on the stove over low heat and mix in 400 g shredded cooked chicken (the first half of the second chicken) and a handful of peas. Cook for a further 5–6 minutes. Season and allow to cool to room temperature, then store until use. Upon reheating, add lemon juice to taste and dress with chopped fresh parsley leaves before serving. (This soup is for Night 3 and can be done after you've eaten your yummy chicken and sweet potato fritters, whilst the kids are tidying up.)

11. *Finish the tacos* – Take the remaining half of the second cooked chicken (400–500 g), shred the meat and place in a container to combine in the tacos. On Night 2, place the shredded chicken on a lettuce cup, place a few chopped tomatoes on top, then finish with a dollop of guacamole. Get the kids to make up their own – it makes it much more fun!

MEAL HOME-DELIVERY

In this age of hyper-convenience there are apps and services that could facilitate a life of watching Netflix in bed, requiring you only to have to get up to answer the door. Depending on your location, it's plausible to get your groceries delivered, along with your favourite takeaway foods. As alluring as that may sound, and even necessary from time to time, it's not a long-term solution.

That being said, there are some companies out there that design their meals based on current scientific research and offer 'keto friendly' options within their range. So, I'm not saying avoid home-delivered meals; rather, be selective! Choose ones that haven't doused their food with additives, glutens, sugar and chemicals to extend their shelf life.

SUMMARY

Just to reiterate, there isn't a quick fix to good health. If I had the magic bullet to share with you, I would be writing this from my 80-foot yacht whilst cruising the Greek Islands and not from my bedsit in my tattered underpants. (I'm kidding, I'm in the library . . . in my tattered underpants.) The bottom line is that it takes discipline and planning to keep on track. Equally, it's not the end of the world if you eat a meal that sits outside the lower-carb protocol, and it certainly doesn't 'un-right' the good you've done. There would be no sense in throwing the towel in if your best friend cooks you a delicious pasta dish. The aim is to be as mindful as you can until eventually your decisions become second nature.

For a few years, in my effort to maximise good health I was pedantic about which foods I consumed. Anyone who was around me at this time would tell you I was complete pain in the arse! Eating out in cafés, restaurants and peoples' homes was an activity accompanied by a ton of annoying questions for the barista, waiting staff, chef or friend . . . swiftly followed by eye rolls from friends in my company. I'm the first to admit that I became obsessive. I had created strongly defined parameters that denoted which foods were IN and which were OUT. I still have these parameters, but my attachment to them is not as strong, and hence the regret and guilt associated with eating foods that are OUT has diminished. Essentially, I have softened my grip a little.

My tolerance to foods that are OUT still fits into the 'real food' paradigm — I don't make a habit of eating pizza and doughnuts, but I don't go into a tailspin if I have a higher-carb meal or eat a little cheese from time to time.

If a low-carb approach is new to you, you may need to employ a strategy or two to ensure success. It will be challenging at times, and expect to fall off the wagon, but don't throw in the towel if you do fall off once or twice — your body and mind will love you for it in the long run.

If you've had a lifelong love affair with carbs then it will be tough, but you *can* do it, particularly if you employ some of the strategies listed here. Until your body takes the necessary steps to up-regulate certain pathways for you to become an efficient fat-burning machine, you will experience cravings and mood disruptions. As I've stated, it'll take a day or so to get into ketosis — that's the easy part — but becoming fat-adapted can take a little longer.

Eating a high-carb diet elicits a hormonal response, as we've discussed. This in turn sends a signal to your brain telling you that you're hungry soon after eating. This is a vicious cycle. The hunger signal will still be present for a few days for some, or weeks for others, as you transition. Then there's eating for comfort, which we've also discussed. Carbs signal the reward centre in our brain, something that fats don't really do. So, not only are your hormones making this transition hard for you but the addiction to the neurotransmitter, dopamine, will drive cravings.

What all of this is leading me to say — again! — is: expect it to be hard.

Chapter Six

The macro breakdown

We have all heard of the three macronutrients — carbohydrates, fat and protein — but do we know enough about them? The following chapter is dedicated to getting under the bonnet, getting our hands dirty, and well and truly breaking down each macronutrient. Putting each macro under the microscope is just another step towards making well-informed choices about your nutrition.

Okay, just as a reminder, we are aiming for a macronutrient split of 75:15:10 (fat : protein : carbohydrate) and adhering to the modified keto diet — arguably somewhat easier than the classic keto diet. Let's look at each macronutrient in more detail, looking at daily intake, sources and benefits.

PROTEIN

Where to start? Much revered in the fitness world and much maligned by non-meat eaters, protein is a contentious macro, to say the least, with animal grazing blamed in part for global warming and animal protein blamed for cancer and heart disease. It's not my place to talk about the ethics of eating meat — I've learned over the years that there are certain topics, such as politics and religion, that are entrenched in personal opinion, and the decision to eat meat or not is definitely one of these topics. So, if you *do* decide to eat meat then I'd like to share some recommendations around daily intake, sources and anything else that springs to mind.

Plants also offer protein that is arguably less contentious than animal sources. In fact, most food will have a macronutrient split of some value – meaning it will contain a proportion of each.

Daily intake

Eating too much or too little protein will have health implications. In the past, some children on a classic keto diet experienced stunted growth simply because, in a bid to meet the daily requirements of fat, their intake of protein was sub-optimal. To calculate your optimal daily intake of protein, follow this formula:

1 gram of protein for every kilo of lean body tissue

If you're unsure what your lean tissue value is, then either have a DEXA scan (a body composition scan – see page 64) or go online and estimate your own body fat percentage by comparing yourself to people who have similar body fat percentages. Once you have that figure, apply this formula:

$$\text{total body weight (kilograms)} \times \text{body fat (\%)} = \text{amount of fat mass (in kilograms)}$$

Subtract this number from total body weight = total lean tissue.

Excess protein

We have calculated how much protein is ideal in a day, but what happens if you exceed that amount? Does the extra protein get used for muscle and soft tissue repair/growth? Sadly not! Let's take a quick look at the mechanisms at work when your body has protein intake beyond its physiological requirements.

GLUCONEOGENESIS

If you've never come across this word before, by simply breaking it down into its three parts you'll gain a clue as to its meaning. 'Gluco' refers to glucose, 'neo' means new, and 'genesis' means creation. So, gluconeogenesis is the creation of glucose from new (non-carbohydrate) sources. Through the process of gluconeogenesis your body can convert protein into glucose.

As discussed in Chapter Three, the role of insulin is to transport glucose in the blood into the cells to help maintain healthy blood glucose levels. The hormone batting for the opposition in this scenario is called glucagon. Glucagon stimulates the liver and kidneys to convert protein into glucose, therefore pushing glucose back into the bloodstream and making it available for energy consumption. The relationship between insulin and glucagon is symbiotic; the two hormones dance a merry dance in an attempt to keep blood sugar levels at a healthy level.

When protein intake is in excess of physiological requirements, gluconeogenesis can actually stall or prevent you from going into ketosis. By converting protein to glucose, your body will use this in preference to ketones. So even if you're ticking most of the boxes for the keto protocol — i.e. low carb and high fat — but are eating excessive amounts of protein, you might be compromising your ability to capitalise on the therapeutic ketones.

PROTEIN AND 'SPRING-CLEANING'

Protein can have an impact on insulin, too. Out of the three macronutrients, though, it's little surprise that carbohydrates have the greatest impact. On a calorie-by-calorie basis, carbs have the greatest impact, with protein second and fat last. However, there are some exceptions — certain proteins do stimulate large amounts of insulin.

Excessive consumption of protein can also prevent your cells from 'spring-cleaning', thereby promoting ageing and being detrimental to general wellbeing. I will talk about this in more depth later in the book, but for now let's have a quick look at how too much protein can be detrimental to wellbeing.

I'm sure many of you will have heard of a 'cleanse'. Maybe you've done one yourself, or had a friend or colleague do one. There are many types of cleanses out there — some pedestrian, others just plain weird — but the prevailing reason people undertake a cleanse is always the same. It's to allow the body to 'reset' on a cellular level. The most successful cleanse will include abstinence from substances or activities that cause inflammation, including booze, toxins and high-intensity exercise.

Once things have dialled back or 'simplified', if you like, then the body initiates a metabolic pathway that facilitates the cleanse. The body essentially performs a spring-clean of your cells, removing accumulated debris, including damaged cell components and toxins. This is paramount for wellbeing and anti-ageing. This important process is inhibited by poor diet, poor lifestyle and/or excessive inflammation from exercise. With impaired ability to spring-clean, toxins and damaged components linger and emit pro-inflammatory molecules.

INTRODUCING mTOR (MAMMALIAN TARGET OF RAPAMYCIN)

Well, that rolls off the tongue nicely . . . not.

I touched on this in the previous chapter very briefly, along with its role in inhibiting the 'cleanse' or 'detoxing' of a cell. As you may remember, it's an energetic pathway that is defined as anabolic (building) and stifles removal of dead cell components.

How does mTOR relate to protein? Of all the nutrients that stimulate mTOR, amino acids (protein) top the charts. Eating large amounts of protein (the case for many Westermers) is a sure-fire way to stimulate mTOR and by doing so one of the quickest ways to suppress cellular and mitochondrial 'spring-cleaning' (autophagy). This inhibition prevents your body from removing debris and damaged cells.

Eating the correct amount of protein will help with insulin sensitivity, reduce the signs of ageing and assist with weight management. Calculating your protein intake will become second nature over time. It's safe to say that all us meat-lovers eat too much protein, so perhaps start to monitor the quantity and frequency of your protein intake. Once you have calculated your ideal protein intake (see page 75), I think you'll be quietly surprised by how little it takes to hit the magic number. My advice is to be selective about how many barbecues you go to this year! The general rule is to make your protein serving the size of a small fist. Also, when reading labels, look for *net* grams (because a 220-gram rib eye doesn't equate to 220 grams of protein).

Consuming the *adequate* amount of protein will mitigate the stress placed upon insulin and glucagon and also help you utilise ketones when in a low-carb state.

Satiety

It is well established that proteins and fats are far more satiating than carbohydrates. In other words, they keep us feeling fuller for longer. The mechanism for this is largely due to protein and fat having a reduced impact on insulin, as we've discussed. Carbohydrates, especially high GI versions, can leave us feeling hungry 30–60 minutes after eating a meal, due to the hormonal response that follows.

Once fats, and to a lesser extent proteins, make up the majority of your daily calorie intake, you'll notice a dramatic down-regulation in your hunger signals. This is not to say you won't feel hunger from time to time, but compared to being on a high-carb diet, the hardship is minimal. Eating a higher-fat diet will help to stabilise your blood sugars and actually improve insulin sensitivity, which will help to normalise your hunger hormone, gherlin. Protein sends a strong message to the brain that you are 'done' — and so it's hard to overeat on protein in a single sitting. Eating protein with fat is the recipe for feeling greatest satiety.

I know, personally, my desire to eat has diminished since adopting a higher-fat protocol. I regularly fast (once or twice a week) and believe the only reason I can do this, and do it with ease, is a direct result of my macronutrient choices. Engaging in weekly fasts for 16 hours or so would be much harder on a high-carb diet, with my hormones emitting (screaming!) signals for me to eat.

Don't get me wrong, I love food and I love cooking, so I haven't engineered this protocol in order to save me time and to avoid the 'hassle' of cooking. It's just a protocol that I believe is more aligned with how we are naturally supposed to eat. In other words, eating the types of foods as our ancestors would have, and with similar frequency.

Sources of protein

I grew up in pubs in and around London. My folks focused on food, enticing customers with delicious, comforting, home-cooked food. This wasn't the convention for the time (the mid '70s and '80s). It was my dad who exposed me to the more 'unusual' cuts of meat — beef cheeks, liver, kidney, oxtail, osso bucco. He absolutely loved these meats for their flavour and texture. I'm incredibly grateful to him for the exposure he gave me, for a couple of reasons.

The first is that organ meat is some of the most nutrient-rich foods on the planet. If there was an Olympic Games for nutrient-dense foods, organ meat would be up there on the podium, along with herbs/spices and algae. Meats such as liver, kidney and heart are rich in folic acid, iron, selenium, copper, Co Q10, vitamin A and B vitamins. Remember how I earlier described food as being 'information' for our body? The information from organ meats fosters good health, in contrast to highly processed foods which are often riddled with 'information' that is anti-health. In a perfect world we should get our nutrients from a broad range of food sources, to ensure the broadest range of information. In this scenario your body will have the necessary macro- and micronutrients to optimise health and performance and minimise inflammation and disease. So, to me, organ meat is part of this landscape — just another option for information-rich foods.

If organ meat is mildly confronting to you or your kids, don't feel you have to serve up an entire bowl of brains or a plate of liver and onions. At first, try to incorporate some organ meat into a dish that is a favourite with the family. Adding a little kidney to a bolognese, or some liver to a burger patty, is a great starting point. Generally speaking, organ meat has a distinct flavour, so adding a *little* to a crowd-pleasing recipe won't disrupt the recipe hugely but will get you and your family accustomed to the flavour. They might not even notice, in which case you've added value to their meal with no resistance.

There are plenty of organ meat recipes in this book and on my websites, so start experimenting when the time is right.

The second reason I'm grateful for having been exposed to underappreciated cuts of meat concerns respect for the animal. I completely understand that eating meat isn't for everyone, but I think that if you *do* choose to eat meat then you should be open to eating 'nose to tail', not cherry-picking the sirloin or eye fillet. Eating nose to tail will minimise animal wastage.

Another recommendation I want to throw in at this point is to consider buying alternative cuts, ones that offer you valuable nutrients from the connective tissue, such as gelatine, collagen and glucosamine chondroitin — all important 'information' for soft tissue repair and growth. These cuts, which often still have the bone attached, require long, slow cooking. Examples are osso bucco and lamb shoulder.

Cooking meat with bones/connective tissue attached typically means a cut with more fat, too. Next time you're at your butcher, have a look at a lamb shoulder — it *should* have a layer of fat on it. Obviously you can have this removed by the butcher, but in the interests of a higher-fat protocol, I'd suggest leaving it on. It's the fat and connective tissue that will add flavour and mouth-feel to the dish.

Grass-fed versus grain-fed

Much has been said in recent years about the superiority of grass-fed animals over feedlot animals, from health and ethical points of view. Once again it comes down to preference, availability and affordability. For me it comes down to choosing an animal that has lived a life with as little distress as possible: an animal that has been able to roam relatively freely, has not had antibiotics or growth hormones injected into it, and has eaten food that mimics its choice were it a wild animal. In an age of industrial farming, having all these boxes ticked can be a challenge, but you can always ask your butcher if you're unsure. Grass-fed animals tend to produce more nutrient-dense meat, milk and fat.

CARBOHYDRATES

Hopefully by now I've communicated that not all carbohydrates are created equal. Sure, there are similarities in terms of their composition, but they can be vastly different in relation to the 'information' they hold. Some carbohydrates promote health and longevity, others the antithesis of this. This alone makes it very confusing.

Veggies

First, let it be understood that by no means am I prescribing a low-carb diet that excludes veggies and fibre. In fact, quite the opposite. Your diet should include an *abundance* of veggies . . . because veggies *are* carbohydrates! (Sorry if that seems blindingly obvious but it isn't common knowledge. For some people, carbs are represented solely by pasta, rice and potatoes.)

The key to success is to limit the number of starchy and/or high glycaemic veggies consumed, such as sweet potatoes and yams, as well as refined carbs such as pasta. The low-carb veggies are the ones that we can welcome with open arms.

Veggies that will be your friends in your pursuit of health and longevity include:

asparagus	cauliflower	mushrooms
aubergine	celery	onion
avocado	chard	pak choi
broccoli	courgettes	peppers
Brussels	cucumber	rocket
sprouts	garlic	spinach
cabbage	kale	tomato

Fruit

We haven't talked about fruit all that much in this book. We did mention earlier that fruit is perennial these days, as opposed to seasonal, which was the way our ancestors experienced it. The modern-day year-round availability of fruit can do us a disservice. Although completely 'natural', fruit does contain sugar, and some fruits are super-glycaemic, so we do need to be mindful of fruit consumption. I like to think this book is not dogmatic or prescriptive, but I will say, please reconsider drinking fruit juices! Whether freshly squeezed or store-bought, the process of extraction has stripped the fruit of its natural 'sugar buffer', fibre. Fibre slows the rate at which sugar can be absorbed in the gut and lowers its GI.

Fibre

Fibre is essential for health — it's used as food by the bacteria in our large intestine and is a necessary part of fostering an optimal gut microbiome. Insoluble fibre, as the term suggests, passes through the body undigested, whereas soluble fibre is converted to short-chain fatty acids. It's the short-chain amino acids that nourish your healthy gut microbes and are used as fuel for your cells.

Fibre also acts as an anti-nutrient, meaning it slows down the absorption rate of carbohydrates, reducing the spike of blood glucose and insulin. Insoluble fibre also forms a 'mesh' in your intestine, soluble fibre then plugs the holes — collectively helping to protect the gut.

Pulses, legumes and other higher-carb foods

Pulses and legumes are valuable sources of fibre, which has many beneficial properties, as described above, but they contain a great deal more carbohydrates. The higher-net carb value doesn't rule them out altogether, but it does mean they'll need limiting if the goal is ketosis.

Some sources of higher-carb foods include banana, beetroot, buckwheat, kidney beans, potato, quinoa, sweet potato, taro and yams. This list doesn't include any refined foods — all the foods in the list are natural and fit into the hunter–gatherer protocol — *but* they have more net carbs than is necessary, given that our aim is to be in ketosis. Equally, I'm not suggesting that they are on the banned substances list. (You do not have to cross the road if confronted by a banana!) But being mindful of the net carb value of foods is a great place to start in a bid to secure a path to optimal health and performance. Alternatively, include the above foods but acknowledge the volume (quantity). You'll need to drastically restrict quantities to meet the low-carb protocol.

For instance, a baked potato will yield approximately 54 grams net carbs. If our aim is to secure less than 40 grams of carbs per day, having a baked potato for lunch has exceeded your carb intake for the *entire* day. Not the end of the world, clearly, but for optimal health and performance, aiming for a low-carb protocol is ideal. That being said, if you live for baked potato, simply adjust the volume to fit into the protocol.

•

I have an imaginary friend, Debbie. I've been talking about and referring to her for years now! Debbie represents someone whom I'm hoping to reach and help with my protocol. She is around 35, has two kids and lives in a large country town. She hasn't paid particular attention to her health for most of her life, but as she's grown older she's been trying to be a little healthier and impress this upon her kids. She is a stay-at-home mum and doesn't have bundles of cash to splash out on health products. Since her early 30s, she has put on weight, developed some daily aches and pains, and suffers from a lack of energy and brain fog.

Debbie wants to make better choices but as you can imagine, googling 'best diet' or 'workouts' would present a mix of opinion, many of which would conflict. Debbie motivates me to make the protocol easy to follow.

Over the years I've had countless conversations with friends, family members, fellow parents at school and audience members at various talks and demos I host about optimal nutrition and the path to health. There is a sentence that I wish I'd had a dollar for every time I've heard it and it goes something like, 'That's all well and good, Scott, but doesn't it just come down to everything in moderation?'

The 'everything in moderation' approach is one potentially riddled with pitfalls. It's not to say it can't work, but with so many variables and different base levels it's not a one-size-fits-all solution. It's an approach that has given many of us in the Western world a little 'out', if you like — one that could be stopping us reaching our greatest health potential.

Base level

The 'everything in moderation' rule might be workable if your base level of health is good and is reflective of the foods you embrace **most** of the time. In other words, if you eat healthily 90 per cent of the time but occasionally have foods that aren't healthy, then you can argue that this might not have a huge impact on your health. But, as the percentage declines and more of the naughty food prevails, the balance begins to tip. My stats, for example, might be 95 per cent healthy food and 5 per cent not healthy — a tolerance that my immunity, gut and mitochondria can arguably handle. But for someone who eats healthily 50 per cent of the time and the remainder is unhealthy, then that will have a far more detrimental impact on health.

Debbie eats healthily 60 per cent of the time — doesn't sound too bad, hey!

If she eats three square meals a day, over the course of a week that equates to 21 meals (not including snacks and drinks). Of which 12.6 meals are healthy and 8.4 are unhealthy per week (60:40). Over the course of a year that equates to 655.2 healthy meals and 436.8 unhealthy meals. Debbie might live to 80 years old.

This works out to be 34,944 unhealthy meals!!!

I'm not trying to be alarmist but rather bring attention to the fact that the 'everything in moderation' approach might not always serve us, from a health perspective. If we were to pull apart the unhealthy meals that Debbie has been having, we'd see that they'd contain unhealthy fats including artificial trans fat and high levels of omega 6 and high sugar. Later in this chapter I mention how reactive and unstable these fats are and how sugar can affect gut health and inflammation. These two factors alone can lead to damaged cell walls, damaged mitochondria and DNA, stress, inflammation and compromised immunity. If this is happening as a consequence of 8.4 meals per week and 436.8 meals a year, it is a large burden on her overall health.

The underlying message is to embrace foods, macronutrients and a lifestyle that minimises inflammation — which is the cornerstone of disease. Every morsel that passes your lips is either healthful 'information' or not — the more of the healthful information we give our body, the healthier our gut, mitochondria, immunity, mood and cognitive function will be.

If we know that sugar and processed oil promote inflammation, it's comforting to know that elevating ketones in the blood (ketosis) acts as signalling molecules which have an effect on inflammosones ('multiprotein'), which promote inflammation in our body. Ketones inhibit the activation of inflammasomes — which would otherwise release inflammatory incytokines. This mechanism helps to minimise the age-related diseases associated with systemic inflammation, and signals for genes to be turned on that promote health and longevity.

•

Debbie is not too different from most of us. She is trying to look after her health some of the time, but she knows she could do more. Recently she has begun keeping a food diary to get an idea as to what she eats on any given day. Let's have a look at her food diary for the last 24 hours.

Breakfast:
cereal — 69 g net carbs
2 slices of toast — 22 g net carbs
juice — 25 g net carbs
latte — 9 g net carbs

Lunch:
ham and salad sandwich — 35 g net carbs
soft drink — 36 g net carbs

Dinner:
pizza — 22 g net carbs
ice-cream 15 g net carbs

Total: 233 g net carbs (This is significantly high, but it's arguably a common value in a Western diet.)

We know that Debbie eats unhealthily 40 per cent of the time and would benefit from reducing her daily net carb intake. If this was typical of Debbie's diet, then she has much to gain from the low-inflammatory benefits that a low-carb diet will elicit. In order to benefit from being in ketosis, Debbie should aim for 30–40 grams net carbs daily. In terms of transitioning, her challenge would be to create new habits around selecting more appropriate carbohydrates.

The potato paradox

You wouldn't necessarily think potato could feature in a low-carb approach to nutrition – however recent findings have identified that heating and cooling of white potato increases its resistant starch and lowers its carb value. These values increase and decrease respectively for every subsequent reheat and cooling. An interesting, fun fact for every potato-lover out there!

Resistant starch

Just to throw a spanner in the works, as briefly mentioned there are a bunch of veggies that don't fit in the low-carb category but which have valuable resistant starch. This starch acts as a prebiotic for the gut bacteria. Veggies in this category include: garlic, green bananas, Jerusalem artichokes, leeks, lentils, onions, peas, raw white potato starch (supplement) and white beans.

As I've said before, fostering a healthy gut microbiome is paramount to our health. I'd suggest eating some of the foods in the above list periodically in order to get some of that beneficial resistant starch. Resistant starches are ones that avoid digestion in the upper digestive tract and make their way to the large intestine where our microbes live. Keeping our microbes fed and happy will help us to protect our gut lining, reduce systemic inflammation, manufacture vitamins and produce neurotransmitters.

This might sound weird, but I routinely take raw garlic, Jerusalem artichoke and turmeric as natural 'supplements'. I literally chop them up and swallow them as you would a capsule or tablet. More on these supplements later.

In summary

Carbohydrates are *not* the bad guys, it's simply a case of being selective around which ones to fill your plate with.

- Aim for less than 40 grams net carbs daily
- Reduce refined carbs (rice, bread, pasta, cakes, doughnuts, etc.)
- Eat low-carb veggies in abundance
- Incorporate resistance starches
- Make veggies the hero of your plate and protein the 'condiment'

FAT

I've always maintained that if the macronutrient fat had another name we wouldn't be in the current health predicament we are. The simple fact that it has the same name as a term used to describe being overweight is, and has been, a sticking point for a long time. Maybe we should run a global competition to rename fat as a macronutrient and see if it has an impact on dietary fat consumption in the future? Just a thought.

Let's unpack fat

Fats consist of a group which includes triglycerides, fatty acids, phospholipids and sterols. They have commonality within their structure and physical property — for instance, all fats are hydrophobic, meaning not water soluble.

There are two types of fat, saturated and unsaturated. Of the unsaturated fats, there are sub-types. These are:

1. *monounsaturated*
2. *polyunsaturated*
3. *trans fat*

Let's have a quick look at the structure of fat (triglyceride).

A triglyceride is a bond between one glycerol unit and three fatty acid chains. Fatty acids are long chains of carbon atoms and hydrogen atoms, with some carbon atoms linked to single or double hydrogen bonds. It's the type of bonds in the chain that will determine which type of fat it is.

Saturated fat is characterised by all of the carbon atoms being saturated with hydrogen atoms. They do not contain double carbon bonds. Saturated fats are typically solid at room temperature and have a high melting point. They include butter, beef dripping and coconut oil.

Unsaturated fat is characterised by at least one double-bonded carbon atom. The double bond can take on one of two formations. These will ultimately determine whether it's a trans fat or another type of unsaturated fat (monounsaturated or polyunsaturated).

Trans fats occur when the hydrogen atom appears on the opposite side to the double-bonded carbon atoms. Trans fats are solid at room temperature and have a high melting point. There are naturally occurring trans fats that appear in dairy and meat, primarily (ruminant fat), and industrial versions which are added to fast food and some baked items. These are best avoided. When you're reading your food labels, look out for trans fat or partially hydrogenated oil.

Monounsaturated fat is characterised by a single double-bonded carbon atom. The attached hydrogen atoms are on the same side on the double-bonded carbon atom. Monounsaturated fats are liquid at room temperature. They include olive oil, olives and avocado.

Polyunsaturated fat is characterised by more than one double-bonded carbon atom. The attached hydrogen atoms are on the same side. Polyunsaturated fats are usually liquid at room temperature but solidify when chilled. Polyunsaturated fats can be broken down into their omega number: 3, 6, 7 and 9. Omega 3 and 6 are considered essential, as we can't manufacture them ourselves and require dietary intake. The placement of the double-bonded carbon atom in the fatty acid chain will denote which omega it is.

Monounsaturated fat

Omega 3

Polyunsaturated fat

Omega 6

Saturated Fat

Trans fat

Considering this eating plan is suggesting a higher fat intake – in the realm of 75 per cent of daily calories – it's necessary to have an understanding of the different types of fat and, importantly, which ones to embrace and which to avoid. Choosing the 'wrong' type of fat could easily steer you off course and present you with a bunch of health problems. The key is to limit the amount of inflammatory fats/oil – the ones present in highly processed oils and trans fats.

It can be a minefield when first starting out – one that will require the examination of food labels. But just to make things easier, industrial or processed fat/oils are typically found in commercial salad dressings, mayonnaise, peanut butter, canned fish, deep-fried items, crisps, bread, commercial snacks and baked goods . . . Basically, most items on the supermarket shelves!

When you're reading labels, look out for these key words:

rapeseed oil
peanut oil
cottonseed oil
grapeseed oil
sunflower oil
safflower oil
trans fat
hydrogenated fat

The oils listed above have high levels of omega 6. This is the issue.

HIGH OMEGA 6

Before we explore the risk associated with omega 6 fatty acids, we need to first acknowledge that they are essential fatty acids – meaning we *need* to consume them. A diet devoid of omega 6, or 3 for that matter, would lead to a string of health problems. Conversely, health problems arise when the quantity of omega 6 starts to blow out. As we can see from the list of foods above, it's incredibly easy to ingest excessive amounts of omega 6 on a typical Western diet. Another important variable is the ratio between omega 3 and omega 6. Both are essential fats, but when the ratio starts to blow up in favour of omega 6, health issues will ensue.

We've established that polyunsaturated fats (omegas 3 and 6) contain more than one double-bonded carbon atom along the fatty acid chain.

These double bonds are highly susceptible to oxidation — meaning that exposure to air will damage the fat — and it's the damaged (oxidised) fats that cause stress within our bodies. Similarly, when these types of fats are exposed to pressure, heat or UV light, they will oxidise (damage) the fat. Consider the damaged fat as being volatile or reactive, causing stress and inflammation to our cells.

I strongly urge you not to consume these reactive oils. As you embark on this low-carb/high-fat protocol, make sure you read food labels. I can't stress this enough, for the prevalence of harmful vegetable oils is astonishing. A rule of thumb would be to lower your consumption of omega 6 and increase your consumption of omega 3, either through supplementation or through marine sources (fish and krill). A primary objective of this protocol is to minimise the disruption of your cells, and in particular your mitochondria. Processed vegetable oils are just one of the contributing factors that can lead to disruption of mitochondria. Damaged mitochondria produce reactive oxygen species, or ROS, which in turn can damage DNA, leading to cell mutation and cancers.

•

Okay, so we have looked at the fats to eliminate in our quest for good health, now let's look at some of the fats that are considered healthy and will contribute to being in ketosis. In order to obtain 75 per cent of your calories from fats, start to become acquainted with the fats listed below.

Animal fats

Animal fats from grass-fed sources are higher in omega 3s than conventional fat. The absolute amount isn't very high, but if you eat a significant amount of animal fat — as many people on 'primal' diets do — the omega 3 adds up. Grass-fed fat is also higher in antioxidants, making it more resistant to oxidative damage during cooking. Pastured animals allowed to eat fresh grass and forage for wild herbs will effectively produce antioxidant-infused meat with greater oxidative stability than animals raised on concentrated feed.

Coconut oil

Coconut is one of nature's superfoods. It is anti-microbial, anti-viral and anti-fungal, meaning it helps fight pathogens and viruses, but is also a great source of fat. It will double up as a moisturiser and has in-built UV protection if you get caught short out in the sun (although I wouldn't recommend staying out for too long — it's hardly factor 30).

Most of the fat in coconut oil is medium-chain triglycerides, which means this can be rapidly transported to the liver and once there converted into ketones. Ketones are then pumped into the bloodstream and become available for energy.

Try cooking more with coconut oil; it copes well with high heat and is very stable. It's possible to add coconut oil to your tea or coffee as an easy way to get healthy fats into you . . . and a way to propagate production of your ketones. From a flavour perspective it doesn't always lend itself to certain cuisines — Italian, for instance. But experiment and see what dishes it suits. I add it to most Asian dishes when cooking at home.

MCT oil (C8 and C10)

MCT oil (medium-chain triglycerides) is a more concentrated version of coconut oil. In fact, MCT is typically derived from coconut oil (sometimes palm oil too) and can be bought at health-food shops and even in some major supermarkets now. 'Medium chain' denotes that there are 6–12 carbon bonds in the fatty acid chain (there are also short-chain and long-chain fatty acid chains). MCT is a clear, tasteless oil, which makes it ideal for incorporating into drinks and sweets, or taking off the spoon. The benefit of medium-chain triglycerides is that they can bypass the usual digestive process for fats and instead go directly to the liver, via the hepatic portal. Once in the liver they are rapidly converted to ketones and released into the bloodstream, thence transported throughout the body.

When choosing your MCT at the shops, look for C8 and C10 — caprylic and capric respectively — both fatty acids that will help with ketone production. We touched on MCT a few chapters back but I wanted to remind you of the caveat that comes with taking MCT oil. As your coach I care for not only your health but also your dignity — you'll thank me later! Sometimes your liver cannot deal with the quantities of fat being dumped into it — this can happen when you're consuming MCT straight off the spoon. As a consequence it'll dump it back into your intestine. At this point you can feel a sore stomach and/or a strong desire for a bowel movement . . . and when I say strong, I mean strong! So, to avoid any accidents at home or in the workplace, I encourage you to test your tolerance gradually. Start off with 1 teaspoon a day and over weeks build up to 3–5 tablespoons a day. If and when you feel gut disruption, accept that that might be your upper limit per dose.

Fats from fish

Fish such as herring, sardines, salmon and mackerel are rich in omega 3 (remember we are trying to up our omega 3 to support a healthier ratio between omega 3 and omega 6). Fish is also a rich source of EPH and DHA, a precursor to DNA and helpful in maintaining happy and healthy mitochondria — a primary goal of this protocol.

Sardines are a pretty inexpensive food. If you buy them tinned, make sure they are in olive oil or water. There are risks associated with getting all your omega 3 from larger predatory fish — namely, accumulation of heavy metals and toxins — so just make sure you include fish in your diet that is from lower down the food chain. Sardines and anchovies are good examples. There is also the ethical consideration of overfishing in waters around the world. I've been privileged over the last four years to work with the Marine Stewardship Council. This is a global governing body that protects fish stocks and is the gold standard for sustainability. So if you're unsure which fish to buy, head to www.msc.org or look out for the blue tick on any packaging.

Eggs

For many years eggs were thrown under the proverbial bus along with saturated fat, and still to this day have a stigma attached to them. The spiel was that eggs contain cholesterol, which would negatively affect blood cholesterol levels. Nowadays it is known that dietary cholesterol has little bearing on health.

The term 'superfood' is one that has been bandied about a great deal in recent years but I believe the humble egg is worthy of this title. Small, compact, affordable, healthy and versatile, it ticks all the boxes. Eggs provide us with the eight essential amino acids and in addition offer protein and vitamins A and E.

Overcooking eggs can negate any health properties, so I recommend cooking your eggs on a low heat and aim for the runny end of the spectrum. I love to slow-cook my scrambled eggs with some butter, then I take them out of the frying pan when they are still a little 'uncooked' and rely on the residual heat to cook them further on the plate. Exposing eggs to high heat can disrupt their nutritional benefits so my tip is cook on a low heat. This applies to boiled eggs, scrambled, poached and fried – cooking eggs on high heat gives you a larger window for error, too. When cooking on a high heat (as applies to all ingredients), you'll have a smaller window in which the food is 'perfect'. It's even possible to eat raw eggs, the risk of salmonella is negligible. If you are pregnant or giving to a child always ensure that eggs are stamped with a red lion if you intend to partially cook them or eat them raw. This shows that they are produced under the British Lion Code of Practice.

Lastly, on the topic of eggs – if you have access to and can budget for free-range or organic eggs then I'd recommend it – they have a much better nutritional profile but also the chickens are kept in better living conditions.

Nuts and seeds

I remember, when I was knee-deep in the paleo diet several years ago, that nuts were a way of life. They are a great source of vitamins and minerals, along with some omega 3s, but there are some small caveats around eating them. Nuts and seeds also contain omega 6 — BUT not all nuts are created equally. There are some nuts that have healthier ratios between omega 3 and 6.

Nuts/seeds (omega 6:omega 3)

The balance between omega 6 and omega 3 in some common nuts and seeds. (Listed in order of best to worst!)

Walnuts 4:2
Macadamia 6:3
Pecans 20:9
Pine nuts 31:9
Cashews 47:6
Pistachios 51:9
Sesame seeds 58:2
Hazelnuts 90:0
Pumpkin seeds 114:4
Brazil nuts 377:9
Sunflowers seeds 472:9
Almonds virtually no omega 3

Data source: Dr Loren Cordain, thepaleodiet.com

You can see as you go down the list that the omega 6 content starts to blow up — with walnuts, macadamias and pecans being the most beneficial. Nuts are incredibly more-ish little suckers so you may require some willpower to limit your intake. Occasionally I'll roast some macadamias in coconut oil and rosemary . . . OMG . . . so good! (See recipe page 249.) I deliberately only make small quantities of these because I know once I start eating I find it hard to put them down . . .

Avocado

More expensive than gold, but incredibly healthy, if you can afford an avo every now and again, go for it. Brimming with monounsaturated fats and antioxidants/vitamins, the avo is definitely up there on the foods to prioritise on this protocol. In my mind, the combination of avo, lemon, sea salt and black pepper is very hard to beat. You can rescue overripe avos by throwing them in with a smoothie or into a dressing. Both will result in a beautifully rich, velvety texture, with all the health benefits as well.

Olives and olive oil

I recently had the good fortune to visit an olive grove in Victoria, Australia and witness first-hand the process involved in making one of the oldest oils known to humans. Olives are chock-a-block full of healthy fats, and should definitely be considered for this protocol. Toss them in a salad, have them as a snack or make into a tapenade. Olive and olive oil contain antioxidants. The antioxidants that olive oil is renowned for can actually migrate to the foods during the cooking process. For instance, if you sauté broccoli in olive oil, the broccoli, once cooked, will contain more antioxidants post cooking than raw.

Butter and ghee

I've had a lifelong love affair with butter. I used to love spreading it on my Ryvitas as a kid. These days I'm happy to cook with it, douse my veggies with it or eat it off the spoon. I often make my own butter at home, allowing me to customise it with various flavours from herbs and spices or simply to salt it with some good-quality sea salt. Making your own butter is super-easy . . . check out my recipes on pages 271–2. Butter from grass-fed cows is rich in saturated fat. In fact, about two-thirds is saturated, with the rest being polyunsaturated.

Ghee is clarified butter. Clarifying is a process whereby the butter is heated. During the heating and cooling process, the fat-rich butter fat separates from the protein, resulting in lactose- and protein-free ghee. Ghee is popular in Indian cooking and is particularly stable to cook with.

Beef dripping, lard and duck fat

Beef dripping, lard and duck fat are fats rendered from beef, pork and poultry respectively. All are a combination of saturated fat, monounsaturated fatty acids and polyunsaturated fatty acids. Obviously they all have slightly different flavours and can bring subtleties to a dish. Don't feel obligated to use the fat of the protein you're cooking with (i.e. dripping with beef or lard with pork). Switching fats with different proteins can elicit some interesting nuances in cooking. All these fats are stable to cook with, and pack a flavour punch. Depending on how friendly your butcher is, he or she may give you some for free, or at the very least super-cheap.

Chapter Seven

Exercise

You may remember that right at the start of this book I let you off the hook, saying I wasn't about to prescribe squats and push-ups. As your coach, I firmly believe you can have great health and strong immunity from nutrition alone – but that's not to say exercise is out the window. Exercise, along with bio-hacks, rest, recovery and smart supplementation, allows you to extend great health to optimal health.

I often think about my imaginary friend Debbie when it comes to exercise. Debbie wants to get fit, because she's been told it's good for her. She goes online and googles 'best way to exercise'. What comes up is confusing, to say the least. Articles on aerobic exercise, anaerobic exercise, low-intensity exercise, high-intensity exercise, walking, CrossFit, weightlifting, Zumba, circuit training and boxing . . . all espousing the amazing benefits of each discipline.

Debbie wouldn't be alone in her confusion. Thousands of people wanting to start a fitness regimen receive a heap of information, some good, some bad, some conflicting, and struggle to reap the benefits of it.

Exercise is a hotly contested area, no different from nutrition, religion or politics – everyone has his or her philosophy and approach. My approach to training is similar to my approach to nutrition. Just as food should be *enjoyed* first and foremost, training or exercise needs to be enjoyed. Failing to tick this box will result in failure to adhere to the exercise plan, long-term. Exercise can lever which genes are expressed and either enhance health or detract from it. Knowing which mode of exercise will benefit us most, as well as the volume and intensity of that exercise, will directly help to maximise health.

It's possible to be fit and simultaneously unhealthy, just as it's possible to be un-trained and healthy.

I know only too well the pros and cons of exercise. I've had a long history of sport and training. As a schoolkid I was in every sporting team. School to me was an opportunity to play sport, and I embraced it wholeheartedly . . . before school, at lunchtimes and after school. I did okay academically, but in sports I excelled. Upon leaving school this love continued and I played high-level soccer and volleyball. In my late 20s and 30s I got into running and competed in many 10-kilometre and half marathons with some success, running a sub 33-minute 10 kilometres at the height of my running career. All my life I've trained and played sports and at every occasion have given 100 per cent.

This approach and mentality helped me win accolades, but I also paid a price. I have experienced serious injuries — big enough to make me re-evaluate how I train. At the age of 13 I was diagnosed with osteochondritis in my knees, a condition affecting the integrity of the joint. I was sidelined from sport and training for 12 months under strict instructions from my doctor. I remember that being one of the longest years in history. I did as I was told, recovered from my injury, then I went on to train indiscriminately as I had done previously.

Fast forward to 2005. At this point I had been running, and running a lot. Most days I'd throw on my sneakers and hit the pavements and parks of Sydney. It became my identity, and I relied on running to elevate my mood, to supply me with the excuse to eat everything in sight, and to keep me 'fit'. (I put 'fit' in quotes here because at the time I was 'fit' but not *healthy*.) The volume and intensity of running I was doing was far from optimal for my health.

In the spring of 2005 I injured my back — an injury that forced me to rethink not only my exercise regimen but my life. For the next seven years I came to terms with the fact that I couldn't train indiscriminately any longer. It was seven years of wrestling with training and inflammation, of re-evaluating identity, of pain, depression and frustration. It was a dark period of my life.

With most dark episodes there are often silver linings, and mine was no different. The whole experience forced me to change jobs. I stepped into the fitness world in 2005/2006, and after realising my attitude to exercise wasn't working for my injury, I radically changed my approach to working out. Both have been positives in my life. The penny also dropped with nutrition. I realised that I needed to look at how nutrition could also support my injury. I started reading on the topic of food and inflammation, and the more I read the more it made sense. The take-home message was this: the foods I consumed could help to minimise inflammation and promote health and recovery. I began to modify my dietary macronutrients and the change was tangible. Now, at the age of 41, I'm healthier than I've ever been, at my optimal weight, injury-free and intrinsically happy. I now want this for you!

Back to Debbie. When she was googling exercise, no doubt she would have come across the claims that exercise burns calories and that this was the solution to weight loss. Movement *will* burn calories, *but* the sooner we drop the belief that exercise is the solution, the better.

YOU CAN'T OUT-TRAIN A BAD DIET

When I first started in the fitness industry in 2005, I thought the epitome of health was reflected in how fit you were. My position was a blend of my exercise science background, in which physiology and performance are the only consideration, coupled with my own interest and desire to be the fittest guy around. Back then I attached a great deal of ego to my training, which pushed me to my limits and helped me become a legitimate competitor. I used to train most days and flog myself, training through pain, tiredness and staleness, which ultimately led to my body breaking down.

When I cast my mind back to those days, I'm the first to say that my obsession with fitness was unhealthy. It's an all-too-familiar scenario that is played out in gyms and fitness centres across the Western world – seeing fitness as the solution to health. I firmly believe we can be lean, healthy and strong from nutrition alone – it's our genotype. Fitness is like the cherry on top.

If nutrition (which accounts for 80 per cent of your health) is neglected in preference of training, then you are, at the very best, spinning your wheels, or in a holding pattern. Most likely you'll be in a negative spiral – therefore the notion we can out-train a bad diet simply doesn't apply. Fuelling your body with 'information'-rich foods is a much better approach and one that doesn't require working up a sweat. Even better!

It's hard for me to prescribe the perfect fitness plan because we are all wired for exercise differently. Having said that, there are some broad brushstrokes we can all adopt to facilitate optimal health. Exercise, if done right, can turn on genes for health, longevity and improved cognitive function. On the flipside, too much exercise can be detrimental to health, so it's about being smart around your training to maximise the health and therapeutic properties. Understanding variability between genders, races and individuals will go some way towards the redundancy in comparing yourself to others – social media can create an environment of comparisons, self-analysis and unrealistic expectations BUT knowing what level of exercise is going to help YOU is the key.

If you are going to get the cherry on top, here are some guidelines . . . but I recommend engaging with a fitness professional to personalise a little more for individual success.

DO SOMETHING YOU ENJOY

This *has* to be the first cab off the rank. There are so many modes of exercise these days, if you look hard enough there'll be something that flips your switch. The gym isn't for everyone; there are plenty of other options. Finding something that you get excited about is the key to success.

Because we aren't looking to exercise as the solution to health, and don't need to flog ourselves to achieve 'success', choose something that incorporates 'play'. By 'play' I mean an activity that is enjoyable in the purist sense — it could be playing frisbee or simply surfing — but something that the 'fitness' element is secondary to the enjoyment of the actual activity. Think about tennis, perhaps, or rock climbing, basketball, CrossFit, gymnastics, dance . . .

BUDDY UP

I've said this before, but buddying up can be incredibly beneficial, particularly if you're just starting out on your fitness journey. A buddy will make you accountable and will help to keep you on track. At the beginning of the week, map out the days/times you intend to train and lock it in the calendar. If you're partial to a few bevvies on a Friday night, schedule your training for Saturday to force you to reconsider those drinks, or at the very least curtail the evening's recklessness. If teaming up with more than one person means a greater likelihood of success, then do it!

WARD OFF AGEING

As we age, changes occur in hormones, and consequently physiology. Exercise can help or retard the speed of change. Typically there will be a decline in muscle density, bone density, endurance and mobility. Engaging in strength-based exercise as we get older is highly recommended.

If the thought of going to a gym is far too confronting, even with a buddy, then don't fret. Strength training can happen anywhere — even in the confines of your living room. Depending on where you are on the fitness spectrum, your own body weight might be sufficient to elicit a strength response. Otherwise, investing in some hand weights or kettle bells might serve you well.

A loss in mitochondria as we age will demonstrate a decline in endurance and output. Exercise manifests as stress to our physiology. In direct response to this stress, our body will adapt to compensate. Generally speaking, the more stress we place upon the body the more adaptations will take place. Through exercise it's possible to retard the decline in mitochondria and actually encourage mitochondrial biogenesis.

In previous chapters we have seen how ketosis promotes mitochondrial biogenesis. Very quickly you can see how exercise can complement diet to improve health and longevity.

INTENSITY

Leaving the gym drenched in sweat, stinking and red-faced is not the solution, to my mind. I'm not advocating that we shouldn't push hard occasionally, but remember that the underlying message with this protocol is to minimise inflammation, and training flat out all the time evokes a hormonal response that is inflammatory. This hormonal response might actually be contributing to fat storage, preventing you from hitting your ideal weight. Less emphasis should be placed on the notion that the harder we work the better the results, for there's a point of diminishing returns. This point will be different for everyone, and changes as we age.

During the post-exercise period there will, depending on intensity, be a period of catabolism (breakdown). This is normal, and a necessary part of training and adapting. Catabolism is followed by an anabolic (building) phase. If you train too soon after the previous session, you will not have recovered fully, and this, repeated chronically, leads to overtraining — which can be very detrimental to health. The harder we train, the longer the period of recovery needs to be.

Training, together with excessive protein (an all-too familiar scenario), will promote the energetic pathway of mTOR — I have mentioned mTOR a few times in this book. It's not necessarily a negative thing, but if this pathway is on constantly due to insufficient rest days then it'll inhibit the 'cleansing' of the cell — which is necessary for health and longevity.

Go hard occasionally but don't copy my mistakes of the past: don't be either 'on' or 'off'. Throw in sufficient rest and recovery. Your own body is often the best indicator of fatigue. For years I used to 'push through' any level of fatigue through pure determination (read: pig-headedness), but these days I choose not to train. There have been days that I've literally done an about turn upon arriving at the gym because my body was telling me to rest. Back in the day, I saw that as a sign to work even harder . . . a sign of weakness, almost. I'd like to think I employ smarter strategies these days and have less ego attached to my workouts. Learning to embrace rest and recovery can often lead to greater results than red-lining the whole time.

VOLUME

This is how often you train and for how long. Volume is intrinsically linked to intensity. As a general rule of thumb, the more intense the exercise, the more rest and recovery you'll need. Just as food is viewed as 'information' throughout this book, exercise ought to be understood as 'stress'. The greater the stress, the more cellular disruption and the greater the need for rest, recovery and supplementation.

An example of this is a CrossFit workout. It might only take 30–40 minutes but it requires every ounce of energy and works every facet of fitness, strength, power, mobility and endurance. Therefore the 'stress' or disruption is greatest. There would be an implicit need to recover adequately in order to perform the next session, and this might mean taking two or three days off training. In contrast, if the same person went for a 20-minute walk then there'd much less need to recover. Volume is greatly dependent on the individual, training history and goals.

BRAIN BOOSTING

Not only can exercise promote the growth and health of mitochondria but it also stimulates brain-derived neurotrophic factors. I mentioned BDNF a while back in relation to ketosis stimulating neuron growth and function. Well, exercise can have a similar effect. Once the protein is stimulated it triggers the growth of neurons in the brain. So diet and exercise combined can help us grow new neurons and simultaneously ward off neurological decline.

STALENESS

Training should never feel dull. If it does then it's necessary to mix things up a little. This can be achieved in a number of ways:

1. Change gyms
2. Get a training partner (someone who you find inspiring)
3. Invest in a new programme
4. Invest in a new modality
5. Train outdoors
6. Read and watch material that will inspire you

SUMMARY

- Incorporate strength training into your regimen
- Work up a sweat

- Ensure adequate rest and recovery
- Stress the body in various ways
- Target strength, muscular endurance and mobility
- Train outdoors from time to time
- Don't red-line all the time

Chapter Eight

Health-enhancing tips and hacks

Great health can be achieved through nutrition alone. To take *great* health to *optimal* health, there are myriad of additional and supplementary tricks, hacks, potions, remedies and practices that will have you feeling the best version of yourself in no time. I'm not suggesting you employ all of them, but perhaps try some. Combined with good nutrition, they will help to clear the brain and body fog, leaving you energised, alert and healthy.

This chapter is devoted to a few hacks that have been shown to optimise health (both physical and mental) and performance. However, it's always advisable to seek guidance from a health-care practitioner beforehand.

Many of the below are non-negotiables for me. I attribute my current health to adhering to a diet that promotes a low-inflammatory environment, but also to the many complementary hacks that contribute to overall health. Broadly speaking, it's about minimising inflammation and certainly preventing systemic inflammation. Once this becomes the primary driver for you and is the motivation to choose certain practices and foods over others, you'll see a huge improvement in your health and happiness. Also in the list are a few nootropic supplements — defined as 'smart' drugs or cognitive enhancers.

MAGNESIUM

Arguably the most important mineral, magnesium is essential to the function of every organ in our body. Taking magnesium as a supplement is something that Great-grandma Jean might not have had to be concerned with. She would have received adequate levels of magnesium through fresh food, but due to industrial farming methods and the decline in soil quality, it now needs consideration.

Aim to get magnesium from foods as much as possible. Foods rich in magnesium include dark, leafy greens such as spinach, nuts, dark chocolate, nuts and seeds. Aim for a minimum of 400 milligrams a day and if using supplements, look for the chelated magnesiums (those ending in -*ate*, such as citrate, glycinate or taurate), which tend to be the best absorbed. I'd aim for two or three times this if you're training regularly or are deficient. If taking capsules isn't your thing, it's possible to apply topical magnesium, absorbing through your skin.

TURMERIC

Known for its potent anti-inflammation properties (in particular its active ingredient curcumin), turmeric can be taken as a supplement in powder or capsule form, as can curcumin. I'd recommend taking the raw, complete version of the plant (turmeric), as you'll be consuming valuable co-factors which will support a multitude of enzyme processes, helping to make the body work efficiently. Just make sure you chop it finely as it can be a little unforgiving on the throat.

That's not where the benefits of turmeric stop. Research has shown it has an impact on brain-derived neurotrophic factors (BDNFs). This, to me, is a prime example of food being information. Maybe I need to get out more often, but this genuinely excites me: the fact that we can consume something that has grown in the ground that not only helps with inflammation but has an impact upon the growth of neurons in our brain. Hippocrates was on the money when he stated, 'Let food be thy medicine and medicine be thy food', but we can now expand on that notion, knowing that certain foods are actually life-enhancing . . . turmeric being one of them!

RAW GARLIC

I'm a huge fan of cooking with garlic, and it forms the base for many of my dishes. I also eat raw garlic most days to enhance my health — in particular it can help reduce the severity and frequency of the common cold due to its anti-microbial and anti-viral properties. There's no trick to it, just simply cut, chop or crush the garlic cloves (1–3 at a time) and let it sit on the chopping board for 60 seconds or so to help reduce the enzyme inhibitors — making the nutrients more bio-available. Grab some water or your smoothie and swallow as you would a capsule. For me it's an affordable and easy little hack to boost immunity.

MCT OIL

I've mentioned MCT oil a number of times throughout this book. This reasonably affordable product will help you propagate your ketone production. MCT oil can be bought from health-food shops or ordered online. Being odourless and tasteless, it's ideal for incorporating into drinks and sweets or taking directly off the spoon.

EXOGENOUS KETONES

Exogenous ketones, as opposed to endogenous, are taken as a supplement. The key ingredient is BHB (beta-hydroxybutyrate), which is one of the three ketones naturally produced in the liver. By consuming supplementary ketones you will flood your body with BHB, elevating your blood ketone levels and, according to this definition, putting you into ketosis. This will allow you to reap the benefits of being in nutritional ketosis without necessarily adjusting your food intake. Exogenous ketones are a powerful therapeutic tool but should not replace a nutritionally sound diet (low carb/high fat). Elevated ketones will promote a reduction in inflammation by inhibiting inflammasones, increase insulin sensitivity, normalise blood sugar levels, and provide clean fuel for your brain and heart. Check out my website www.scottgoodingproject.com for information on exogenous ketones.

COFFEE

I haven't always drunk coffee. For years I wrestled with it, loving the taste but not the feeling of slight paranoia that would ensue. After a long hiatus, I'm back . . . and back with a vengeance. I enjoy sometimes three coffees a day now, and use it as a stimulant for both training and work. I'll often time a coffee to coincide with an important meeting, call or event. Caffeine does offer some improved cognitive function, enhanced memory recall and heightened mood.

There is definitely a down side to coffee, though. Excessive caffeine consumption can exhaust the adrenals, leaving you feeling drained. Try a High-octane Coffee (see recipe page 253), a combination of coffee, MCT and butter. It'll help with satiety and the production of ketones.

LION'S MANE

This is a mushroom that can be taken as a supplement. There are products on the market that combine lion's mane with coffee for improved cognitive function. Lion's mane has been shown to influence nerve growth factor, or NGF (a protein responsible for growth neurons), helping to promote the growth and function of neurons. It also enhances cognition by reducing inflammation and improving overall brain health. Lion's mane has been shown to help protect the brain and the cells (axon) by encouraging myelination, which essentially coats your chemical wiring. Myelination helps protect against cognitive decline through ageing, MS, dementia and depression.

CORDYCEPS

Similar to lion's mane, cordyceps is a fungus with potent immunity-boosting properties. It is also possible to use cordyceps as a stimulant, a tonic, and a supplement to increase energy, enhance stamina and reduce fatigue. Again, it can be mixed with coffee for improved mood and focus. In nature, cordyceps acts like a parasite to an insect host. (Don't google cordyceps and ants — you'll never eat them!)

CHAGA MUSHROOMS

Widely accepted as the king of mushrooms, chaga has incredible health benefits. It's not the prettiest-looking mushroom in the forest but is delicious made into a tea or broth. One of the most important things chaga does is activate immune cells called lymphocytes and macrophages. This causes increased production of cytokines. Cytokines are the messengers of the immune system. There are several different kinds, each tasking other cells with specific duties such as organising and rallying white blood cells to fight infection. This stimulation of cytokine secretion creates a more robust immune system that is in a higher state of readiness. Chaga are amazing for boosting your immune system.

REISHI MUSHROOMS

If chaga mushrooms are the kings, then reishi are considered the queens. Reishi is a large dark mushroom with a glossy exterior and a woody texture. Similar to chaga, it contains many health benefits and in particular with fighting allergies, anti-inflammation, anti-HIV, anti-viral and lowers blood pressure. Reishi have long been used in the prevention and treatment of cancers, and they also contain a high concentration of fibre and act as a prebiotic — feeding our microbes.

SAUNA

Exposing the body to high temperatures (above 80°C) is incredibly stressful. The body tries to cool itself, but the extreme temperature exceeds the body's ability to do so, and so the core temperature begins to rise. This is, at the end of the day, stress. But just as exercise is stress for the body, certain mechanisms are initiated to adapt. Cortisol — being our stress hormone — is seen to rise acutely as a response to a sauna, but regular sauna sessions promote a lowering of cortisol.

I've been taking regular saunas since 1998 — that's 20 years of them! For me, they tick a couple of boxes.

One, it gives me **time out**. Sweating it out in a room at 82° Celsius isn't conducive to browsing on my phone. I spend around 45 minutes in the sauna, with a few cold showers thrown in, and it's a period of down time: no communication, alone with my thoughts and a puddle of sweat.

Two, having a sauna has health benefits. A 2015 observational study of 2315 Finnish men showed that men who spent time in saunas were less likely to experience fatal heart attacks. The results showed a strong correlation between the frequency of saunas and protection from heart attacks.

Infra-red sauna

If you find traditional saunas too intense or claustrophobic, another option might be an infra-red sauna. It's not as hot as a regular sauna but is effective at improving health. Mitochondria in your cells use the infra-red light to achieve more adenosine triphosphate (ATP) production — this takes place as the red and infra-red light passes deep into your tissues. Improving mitochondria function is a recurring theme in this book and using saunas to boost mitochondrial function is definitely worth considering.

It's also a vehicle for toxin removal . . . toxins we may have spent a lifetime accumulating. Fun fact (disgusting fact): The infra-red sauna I use supply its clients with white towels; I use one to sit on and one to rest my feet on. After my 45-minute session, the towels are dotted with black marks. It took me a while to cotton on to what the marks are but now know these are heavy metals (toxins) leaving my body and collecting on the towels . . .

GETTING OUTDOORS

When the sun is in contact with the skin, something extraordinary takes place. Einstein discovered, back in 1921, that if we have sufficient levels of DHA (found in omega 3-rich foods such as salmon, mackerel and herring), we are capable of converting the sun's energy into an electric current. This current has an effect on water molecules in the body, which helps to facilitate better hydration and provide fuel for our mitochondria. For more information on healthy levels of sun exposure, see the Cancer Research UK website, www. cancerresearchuk.org

EXERCISE

I know I devoted a whole chapter to this topic, but it's worth a refresh here. Being fit is not a marker of health, *but* being smart about training in tandem with good nutrition, recovery, sleep, hydration and smart supplementation can be a powerful tool. Exercise has a myriad of health benefits, and should be a part of the weekly regimen in a bid for optimal health. I've talked about many things in this book, but certain themes, such as mitochondrial health and inflammation, recur. Smart training — which is the correct volume and intensity of exercise for *you*

– can help to promote the growth of mitochondria and reduce systemic inflammation. Obviously there is an acute inflammatory response to training, but *regular* exercise is seen to contribute to lower systemic inflammation. Low systemic inflammation and healthy mitochondria are two very potent indicators of health and longevity. Seek the advice of a fitness professional to get you on the right track.

COLD THERAPY

I've tried this a handful of times, and have to say it's quite an uncomfortable experience. (I *much* prefer being hot in a sauna.) Cold therapy, or cryotherapy, involves exposing your body to temperatures in excess of −100°C (yes, *minus* 100°C!) for 2–3 minutes. Standing in a pod with socks and gloves on, holding on to my family jewels as the temperature slowly drops, is far from enjoyable – but it's just another mechanism to optimise health, and who said they all had to be enjoyable? Regular exposure to cryotherapy can help reduce systemic inflammation. Exposure to cold temperatures is clearly a stress to the body. In response, the body makes more mitochondria, and this increases your ability to produce energy and burn fat.

SLEEP

Perhaps sleep should have been at the top of the list. Inadequate sleep threatens immunity and gut health, disrupts hormones and promotes fat storage. Good sleep promotes a reboot of our immune system and allows our gut to 'rest' from digesting food matter, not to mention encouraging a decrease in systemic inflammation.

To maximise sleep and optimise health, try the following:

1. Avoid screens for the last two hours of your day prior to sleep. The blue light emitted by devices such as phones and laptops will

interfere with your normal circadian rhythm (your internal body clock) and will disrupt sleep. There are blue light filters you can run on devices these days . . . I suggest you get them.

2. Alternating between hot and cold (finishing on cold) showers will help to promote good quality sleep. How to do hot/cold showers to achieve better sleep:

   - Shower at your usual temperature.
   - Gradually raise the temperature to the point at which it is uncomfortable — ensure your whole body experiences this temperature.
   - Lower the temperature to the coldest possible (no hot tap running) and expose all body parts to this.
   - Raise the temperature again (if you can tolerate a higher temperature than before, do so).
   - Lower the temperature again. Repeat six more times.
   - Start on hot and finish on cold.
   - Only spend time in each extreme temperature for long enough to expose all body parts — particularly the hot shower.

3. Sleep in a cool room (17–19°C). This isn't always easy, but it's definitely worth bearing in mind.

4. Sleep in the dark. I strongly suggest you make your room as dark (and as quiet) as possible to optimise your slumber.

COLLAGEN/GELATINE

There are a number of ways to take collagen or gelatine. Consuming meals using joints of meat that contain these components is one. Ideal meats are osso bucco, lamb shoulder, lamb leg and oxtail. The more connective tissue, the more collagen/gelatine. You can also make or buy bone broth (see recipe page 246).

It is possible to take collagen and gelatine as supplements, too. Gelatine is not soluble in cool water, whereas collagen is — which might make it preferable to gelatine for smoothies, etc. Both are incredibly potent sources of complete amino acids. Both will support healthy hair, nails, tendons, muscles and ligaments. Studies have shown that two aminos — proline and glycine — go directly to areas of trauma for soft tissue repair.

HYDRATION

It may seem blindingly obvious but hydration is a *must*. It's up there with sleep in terms of importance, plus it's free and available nearly everywhere . . . so really, there's no excuse not to stay hydrated. As you transition to a fat-burning machine, by elevating fat intake and reducing carbs you'll naturally reduce the ability of your body to store water (and electrolytes), therefore it's necessary to drink extra . . . plus replace the lost electrolytes by seasoning your food with Himalayan salt or a good sea salt and taking magnesium supplements.

MEDITATION AND MINDFULNESS

I'm not an expert in this area, but I do regularly include meditation and mindfulness in my weekly practice. It took me a long time to let go of the resistance I'd attached to meditation, but now it's simply another facet of my health and wellness package.

How does it benefit me and how will it benefit you?

You'll read more about it in my 60-day protocol, but I'd like to share here my physiological and anecdotal experience. Have you heard of neural plasticity? It's the idea that the brain can change its structure due to different experiences. No longer is there a need to accept that the brain is a fixed structure beyond maturation. Over recent decades, studies have shown that behaviours, thoughts, emotions and experience can positively affect brain development, memory and learning.

Admittedly, most benefits from a plasticity perspective come as a result of dedicated meditation; in other words, you have to clock up some hours to elicit the effects. However, don't let that stop you — a journey of a thousand miles starts with a single step . . . as they say. Meditation or mindfulness, or both, will help to calm you and induce a more rational thought response.

I try to meditate a few times a week and have noticed an improvement in my mood and my ability to handle stressful events. I can now use meditation as a 'touchstone' — if I'm confronted with a stressful event, I can literally tap into an altered state without the need to find a quiet space, close my eyes and focus on breath. It's a potent tool to mitigate stress and therefore inflammation.

Meditation, or even just deep breathing exercises, can also impact health and wellbeing in other ways, including:

- Lengthening of your telomeres — crucial for longevity
- An up-regulation of genes responsible for mitochondrial function, controlling inflammation, energy metabolism and insulin secretion
- Greater resistance to stress
- Improved immunity

DETACH FROM WORK STRESS

In an age of extreme connectedness through a plethora of media, it can be a challenge to switch off from work. I have worked for myself for the past 20 years and am very guilty of always being available by email, text or on the phone, but I know this is sub-optimal for my health. I use certain tools such as meditation, training and the sauna as a means to switch off, but I know I could do more. A stressful work email or call triggers a hormonal response, not dissimilar to the response our ancestors would have experienced on meeting a threat. Some of us experience stress all day, every day. A stressful job, combined with being available at all hours, can lead to a disruption to our hormones, promoting fat storage and systemic inflammation.

I'd recommend creating firm parameters around work – such as only checking emails a few times a day, or not opening your inbox before 8 am and after 6 pm. Easier said than done, I know, but all these little tricks contribute to minimising inflammation and optimising health, longevity and happiness.

•

There are lots of ways to optimise health and stimulate/excite the brain. The key to success is adapting to the protocol over time – there is no right or wrong way to approach it. Some people jump in with two feet and never look back, but for most of us it's a much longer process . . . it was for me! Take small but manageable bites – this is arguably the path to success.

My top tips for Debbie to focus on first would be:

1. Embrace real foods
2. Eliminate processed vegetable oils
3. Improve sleep quality
4. Improve hydration
5. Manipulate macronutrients to suit high fat/low carb
6. Exercise
7. Smart supplementation

With these focuses you're well on your way to optimising health.

Chapter Nine

Case studies

You may remember *waaaay* back in the introduction that I dedicated this book not only to my son, Tashi, but to another little guy by the name of Eli. Odd as it may sound, I've never met Eli, but his story inspired me to contact my publisher to pen this book.

Last year a lady contacted me asking for some recommendations for her son, who was diagnosed with autism at four years of age. I made some broad-stroke recommendations about incorporating more real food into his diet to replace highly processed food and food containing nasties. Eli's mum followed my advice, which supported what she'd read through other sources. She even tried some of my recipes. We maintained communication for months more (and still talk often), and slowly introduced other changes to little Eli's diet, including increasing fat intake and introducing foods that foster gut health.

Nutrition was the cornerstone of the changes we trialled with Eli. However, after several months of witnessing positive results, I suggested Eli try MCT oil (in a bid to curb his sugary cravings and balance blood sugar). The improvements for him were profound. Family members and teachers remarked on the changes, unbeknownst of the modifications made to his diet. Over time we increased his dosage of MCT oil and even tried exogenous ketones. Both produced positive changes for Eli.

One day I asked his mum how well known by other parents in the autism community was the information that she had gathered about nutrition and smart supplementation. Her response inspired me to immediately call my publisher and tell him (in a nice way), 'We *have* to do this book!'

Please meet Bec, Eli's mum.

It was like looking at a 1000-piece puzzle and only seeing the pieces, not the actual picture. After three children I had become less focused on milestones, but by 3½ years Eli wasn't just slower to reach them, he was missing milestones altogether.

Eli was born at 36 weeks. Apart from jaundice and requiring extra feeds, he was healthy. However, by eight months a few bowel issues had turned into severe constipation. There was blood in his stools and he often had stomach cramps. He had gone from breast to bottle (formula) and I had assumed this to be the cause. The maternal health nurse and doctor agreed, and I began to also give water to help with bowel motions.

Over the next few months there was little change, and as he began solid foods, I was advised to wait and see: 'It'll work itself out as he grows.' Coping with his bowels became a daily occurrence and hindered toilet training; however, he had no awareness in that area and I put it down to the bowel.

By 2½ years not only was the puzzle piece of no toilet training there, his speech was also showing signs of delay – he was finding it hard to articulate words and was not even attempting to form three-word sentences. His hearing was fine but he was sensitive to loud noises, and bright or flashing lights startled him to the point of tears. After having his GP again placate me, citing that having older siblings often resulted in speech delays (as older siblings pre-empted needs), I decided to do some research to see if there was any connection between the various puzzle pieces.

Over the course of a few months and seeing different doctors, I had a referral to a speech therapist, who worked weekly with Eli in his home. She too felt that further diagnosis was needed. She had seen first-hand his frustration and meltdowns over various issues, but with her assistance he had begun to form more words, and with the use of some sign language he could communicate basic needs. I was spurred on by his progress and eager to see a paediatrician. I wasn't, however, prepared for the diagnosis of Autism Spectrum Disorder (ASD). Even with a diagnosis I felt I had more questions than answers.

In the weeks following diagnosis I read books and papers on autism, as I felt there was little hands-on intervention information for parents. I wanted to keep up momentum with the progress I'd seen with his speech therapist, through oral exercises and play.

A dear friend, Tracy, had recommended a very unique approach through chiropractic appointments, nutrition and brain gym. We began with two appointments a week. The changes were slow, but you could see through speech and sleep that things were happening for him. By five years and after extensive work with these initial biomedical treatments, Eli was enrolled into kindergarten. He was still not fully toilet trained but he was eager to socialise. I was ecstatic.

Throughout his year at kindy I started to notice the greater role food was playing. He had always been very picky with what he would eat, but due to being invited to parties etc. I noticed how his moods and behaviour would swing, depending on what he ate.

I focused on his diet and saw changes to not just his behaviour and sleep patterns but to his gut and bowel problems. I had another try at toilet training, and in the course of a year we had gained greater control over his constipation and stomach upsets, and he began to use toilets.

In 2016, after assessment, he enrolled into mainstream primary school. It would be five full days a week, so the pressure on his behaviour, focus and toileting was immense. I decided food was going to play a greater role in Eli's ASD management roadmap, but I was unsure to what degree. Throughout his first year at school he missed many days. He would often be tired, emotionally overwhelmed or his gut would become unsettled.

We'd hit another roadblock and his pediatrician suggested this plateau in progress was normal. I wasn't convinced and found an unlikely ally in personal trainer and chef Scott. After sharing our story with Scott, he tweaked recipes and offered advice as to Eli's diet. He suggested reducing sugar and carbohydrates but increasing good fats and protein. Being so selective with foods, the kitchen quickly became a place of experiments, trial and error. Getting Eli involved in cooking meant that he was a little more open to trying new tastes and textures. We reduced dairy products, and coconut milk smoothies became a great way to get more nutrients into him.

As we saw change, Scott suggested we introduce MCT oil. This was the point at which I began to see a change in Eli's focus and cognitive ability unlike I'd seen before with just diet alterations. However, as I was always tweaking his diet, it was hard to see clearly which treatment was having the greatest impact. I didn't care. The combination of utilising wholefoods and supplementation was working to progress his abilities.

I'd love to say we've found the magic key for ASD but I can't. The spectrum is a rollercoaster, often hard and frustrating to navigate. But what I can say is, mainstream treatment in combination with biomedical treatments has provided the strongest and most consistent changes to Eli that I've seen.

The role of real foods to support a wider approach to ASD has given us more control over the rollercoaster.

Real food – and, more explicitly, 'information'-rich food – *has* to be the foundation of anyone's health journey, and this was no different for Eli. I'm not suggesting that a sound diet will eliminate the need for drugs and other therapeutic modalities, but it *will* help to support your immunity and cellular health and minimise systemic inflammation. I understand a great deal of sensitivity is required around prescribing or suggesting a particular approach to nutrition when it comes to parents, but for me it's an affordable, easy consideration to make – one that requires no doctor's prescription, no referrals; just home cooking.

Let me introduce you to Tara. I first met Tara over three years ago when she was working at Fox. At the time I had an idea for a TV show, so we sat down and chatted. She was incredibly invested in her health, and interested in the notion of food being therapeutic. Sadly, the show didn't happen, but I was grateful for the meetings. It gave me an opportunity to make an ally in the industry – someone else who is hell-bent on sharing the potency of real food. Tara was later diagnosed with multiple sclerosis (MS) after lesions were discovered on her brain.

Over to you, Tara.

Reflecting on the first time I met Scott Gooding sums up my life back then. The day we met I was exhausted, had no time for lunch, and from three o'clock I had been itching for a coffee and a piece of cheesecake. I knew we were meeting at a café at 4 pm, so I was ready to place my order and devour my food at first sight. I asked Scott if he would like to join me in a coffee. He politely asked if I could make it a herbal tea. 'Bugger!' I thought. 'He's healthy and fabulous, I can't eat the cheesecake in front of him – but I am way too desperate not to have the coffee.'

Looking back (before my MS diagnosis), my life was chaotic. I was touring a live show internationally, and when I was home

I was either working with other clients or creating new events. It was long hours, eating really badly, drinking too much red wine, and I was the heaviest I had ever been, weighing in at 93 kilos. Sugar was my drug of choice, and I remember waking up one morning, making a coffee, rushing out the door, grabbing two Scotch finger biscuits and thinking, 'Tara, you are eating way too much sugar – you have to stop or it's going to make you sick.'

I went to work that day and was at my computer when a line appeared in my vision. I asked a colleague for some paracetamol, as I thought I was getting a migraine. Over the next day or two the line turned into a black dot that covered three-quarters of a person's face when I looked at them. I went to the ophthalmologist, who told me, after several tests, that the problem was not in my eyes but in my brain.

Reeling, I remember saying, 'BRAIN? LIKE BRAIN-TUMOUR BRAIN?'

He said, 'I'm not sure, we have to rule that out, but we also have to rule out MS.'

I was 45 years old and my life was spiralling out of control: out of control as I lay on an MRI bed while people looked at my brain; out of control finding myself in a neurologist's office; out of control when she told me I had MS and that there was no cure; out of control when the black spot became complete blindness in one eye; out of control when my other eye became painful and doctors started worrying that I would lose vision in that one, too.

MS is a disease that affects 23,000 Australians. With MS, your body's immune system mistakenly attacks and damages the fatty material around nerves in the brain and/or the spine. This material is called myelin. Myelin is not unlike the coating on an electric cord. When someone with MS has a relapse, the immune system attacks the myelin and exposes the nerves that the myelin normally protects, making them malfunction. Depending on what part of the central nervous system is attacked, you could end up with loss of motor function (e.g. walking, hand and arm function), numbness, pain, balance issues, vision changes and changes to thinking and memory. In my case, it hit my optic nerve, resulting in temporary blindness, terrible pain around my eyes, extreme fatigue and a 'brain fog' that left me confused and anxious. I have Relapsing Remitting MS (RRMS), wherein I am prone to a relapse and then periods of remission. In most cases, for those of us with RRMS the disability is temporary. However, for some people it can be permanent.

After six months of struggling, I decided I had to learn how to live with the uncertainty of MS – to find a way to control the uncontrollable. So I looked at the things I could do myself.

First I changed my diet – that seemed the logical place to start. I started researching and found myself exploring diets that avoided foods that could be inflammatory. I also found Dr Terry Wahls's book, *The Wahls Protocol*, and loved her concept of fighting auto-immune disease through nutrition. I started having nine cups of veggies every day.

Then I found doctors who were interested in looking at why my immune system could be overreactive. We looked at everything from the microbiome in my gut to the deficiencies and excesses in my body. I ended up with a personalised regimen of supplementation that gave me what food alone could not.

Within three months my extreme fatigue and brain fog were gone. They have never returned since.

Then I started to exercise; I was so unfit! I started with interval training sessions, and built an exercise programme from there. Now I love to run. If you had told me two years ago that I would be running 8 kilometres regularly, I would have laughed my head off. I exercise without fail five times a week, with a yoga or Pilates session to keep me flexible. This discipline is my way of saying to MS, every day: 'If I can do this, you haven't got me today.' It is so good for my peace of mind.

I also wanted to work on the stress in my life, because I knew that in that arena I was off the Richter scale. So, I learned transcendental meditation. Meditating twice a day for 20 minutes calmed me down; I could feel the difference within a week. I also created some boundaries around my work. I changed the type of work that I was doing and set up a business partnership with a great colleague and friend. It's super-busy, but having a partner means we now share the load. We also have rules around what work we take on.

The weird thing is that this new, balanced approach hasn't had a negative impact on my income. In fact, I am doing better than I was before. Why? I am more focused and things just work better.

The last thing is the most important: I started to love and live my life. Pre-MS I was disconnected from everything but work. Now I make time to enjoy and be really present with my husband, family and friends (no phones!). I do the things I love, like travelling, cooking, riding horses, exercising and taking on projects I am passionate about. I got involved in my MS community to see where I can support others, and learn from those dealing with the same thing. I felt truly supported, healthy and happy for the first time in my life.

So finally, what were the results? Since I have had MS I have never felt better. In 18 months I lost 26 kilograms, going from 93 kilograms down to 67 kilograms. Each time I eat great food I have a strong sense of nurturing my body, connecting me three times a day to the importance of true nutrition.

The way I look at it is that with MS I can still relapse any day. However, if I compare how I live today versus how I was pre-diagnosis, my current lifestyle is a massive asset. I am fitter and stronger (which will be incredibly valuable if I do relapse). What I care about now is that I am appreciating every second of every day, and that gives me the control that MS could have taken away.

PART TWO

My 60-day Keto
Diet Protocol

My promise to you:

- Accessible programme – simple to follow and adhere to
- Simple yet delicious recipes
- All the recipes are gluten-free, refined sugar-free, soy-free, and best of all . . . easy to make!
- As your coach throughout this book, my intention is to simply open the door to a new and improved approach to nutrition and health
- Improved cognitive function
- More energy
- Less 'brain fog'

Your promise to me:

- Open your mind to the protocol – you have nothing to lose
- Be open to new flavours and new ingredients
- No alcohol/drugs during the protocol
- To adhere to the programme. The average person lives for 29,966 days, 60 days is a drop in the ocean!
- No cheat days, in fact, let's take it a step further, no cheat *meals* for 60 days . . . it *can* be done
- When you see and feel the results, tell your loved ones
- The more you put in, the more you'll get out

Introducing my
60-day Keto Protocol

Now you're ready to get started! This section of the book will provide all you need to help you put your new keto and low-inflammation lifestyle into practice. Being in ketosis not only provides your body with an alternative fuel source but is a powerful signalling pathway – stimulating mechanisms for health and longevity. As I've discussed, getting there is one thing, *staying* there is another thing altogether. However, we can all benefit from being in ketosis at some point, or fasting from time to time. Even reducing our refined carb and protein (generally speaking) and increasing our fats and fibrous veggies will promote health.

In Part One I mentioned that one of my key aims with this book is to help you minimise systemic inflammation through a combination of lifestyle and nutrition. My 60-day protocol is designed to take the fuss out of following a keto diet and set you up with a refreshed approach to health. See it as a step-by-step approach – essentially me walking you through the clutter and onto the path to optimal health.

It's important to note that being in ketosis all the time isn't practical for most of us. The idea behind this book is to open the door to an alternative approach — one that also encompasses gut and cellular health. I'd say I'm in ketosis 80 per cent of the time, and can certainly feel the benefits of this. Experimenting with a high-fat/low-carbohydrate diet or fasting will elicit therapeutic benefits but there are occasions when ketosis is not recommended.

There can be instances where being fuelled on fat might not deliver the required energy for certain types of exercise. It's hotly debated, but high-intensity activities like CrossFit or martial arts may not reap the same benefits as lower-intensity activities like distance running. Some people perform well on low carb but others may find their performance hindered. If you're feeling your output is sub-optimal, then try adding some carbs into your post-training feed. You may only need 200–250 grams, but see if that makes a difference. Look to get this from safe starches or gluten-free grains. This is known as cyclic keto . . . low carb on non-training days then upping the carb intake on training days to help replenish cells.

If you follow my protocol to the tee, you should be eating an abundance of veggies; however, people can get carried away with the low-carb side of things. This is more evident when attempting the classic keto (90 per cent fat); in a bid to maximise their calorific intake on fat, veg (carbs) are neglected beyond what is healthy. Even if you attempt classic keto, it is highly recommended that you include fermentable carbs to keep your microbes happy — these resistant starches are found in Jerusalem artichokes, leeks, onion and garlic.

As I touched on earlier in the book, some children who were following a classic keto diet experienced stunted growth due to the inadequate protein intake. This is a consideration, but far less of a risk with this protocol being more aligned with the modified Atkins approach, with a bigger window for protein.

In addition, researchers and academics who promote the benefits of a keto diet acknowledge that changes can occur in lipid profile.

For some people there is an increase in LDL cholesterol and further research needs to be conducted as to the mechanism of this. If your LDL increases, perhaps add additional carbs to the diet, this will help to redress the balance. Check in with your health practitioner regularly to ensure your levels are healthy.

This protocol isn't restrictive – foods that promote a low-inflammatory environment within our bodies are in abundance. Sure, it might mean changing habits but nothing is insurmountable. I've followed it for close to six years with a few tweaks along the way and have never felt more energised in my life. I'm physically stronger than I was at 20 (I'm 41 now), more alert, more resistant to injury and more resistant to illness.

Moreover, I have a good relationship with food. I honestly don't feel I restrict myself with food. I love cooking, which certainly helps me control everything I put in my body – but even when I'm eating out, sure I'm selective, but not restrictive.

I'm not impervious to ageing (shame that!) or work-related stress (work in progress) and I do get sick occasionally *BUT* I feel, based on years of research and personal experience, I've struck on a great solution to health and weight management. It's not a magic potion or pill but rather an approach to food and lifestyle. My primary focus is to care for and nourish my cells, mitochondria and gut health, promoting an environment that is low in toxicity and inflammation. To do this requires some tweaks with foods and macronutrients, along with some bio-hacks. Once you get to grips with the nutrition side of keto, you'll be well on the road to good health. From this point onwards it'll be a case of further optimising your health and performance by including some fitness, some smart supplementation, some daily or weekly bio-hacks – then you'll be a pillar of health inside and out! I'm excited for you!

Preparation is key — the 'On-Ramp' is a necessary part of the journey and is designed to place you in the best possible position to gain maximum benefits.

Store-cupboard cleanse

The first step is to cleanse your store-cupboard and fridge. Please remove any items that will be detrimental to health. The idea here is to remove inflammatory foods and to remove temptation. Store-cupboard swaps are listed on page 64.

The store-cupboard cleanse also includes booze — sorry. For you to truly feel the benefits of this new approach to health, it's important to not cloud your results with alcohol. I'm not suggesting it's off the table forever, but just for a very short period in the scheme of things.

During On-Ramp begin replacing the items in your cupboards fridge and freezer with real food items and staples such as those as listed on page 61. Buy only fresh produce — vegetables, poultry, fish, shellfish, game and offal, and broth up on the healthy fats and herbs and spices. As you adjust to the protocol we can begin to look at other healthy products that come in a packet, but for the On-Ramp, ONLY fresh food please!

Buddy up

This is also an opportunity to recruit allies for your 60-day reset — work colleagues, partner or family. Enlisting comrades will make you accountable to them and them to you. As I've stated throughout the book, the 'transition' phase as you move from high carb/low fat to high fat/low carb can be a little bumpy, which is when having a buddy can really help.

Journal

During the On-Ramp invest in a journal or use the 'Notes' app on your phone – log some commentary on your experiences. Tune into how you are feeling, not just physically, but energetically, cognitively and emotionally. These notes will be your reference point and an opportunity to reflect on your progress. Throughout this 60-day reset you are most likely to experience a decrease in joint aches and pains and in brain fog, and see an elevation in mood, improved clarity and increased energy.

Mindfulness

I haven't spoken about this a great deal throughout the book but it's certainly an aspect that I'd love you to throw into the mix. Mindfulness relates to paying attention to the present moment. Once you're living in the moment, you're not dwelling on the past or worrying about the future. In an age of constant distraction it's so incredibly easy to go an entire day without being in the moment – distracted by traffic, phones, emails, advertising, meetings and life admin.

Practising mindfulness through meditation can have positive ramifications for mental clarity and mindset. By sitting quietly and focusing on your breath or a word (mantra), you are being in the moment. As thoughts come (which is perfectly normal) bring your attention back to your breath or word. It's the act of returning to the focus that is the mindful aspect of it. For years I was resistant to mindfulness simply because I was unsure how to do it, unsure what I should be thinking of or what not to be thinking of when meditating. However, I now understand that it's perfectly normal during meditation to have thoughts that pull you away from the focus and it's simply the act of returning to the focus which is the goal. Over time you'll train yourself to spend more time in the present. Meditation has delivered me some payback in the form of being less reactive and more measured in my responses. It will also help you tune into how you are feeling, which you can record in your journal for further reflection.

A common resistance to meditation is the notion that we don't have enough time in the day, but as a good friend in the industry once said to me, 'Start with one minute a day, Scott!' So that's how I overcame my resistance to it. I literally starting meditating for 1–2 minutes, which has now increased to around 20 minutes a day, and is an integral part of my morning. I reckon we all have at least one minute a day to focus on meditation.

REAL FOOD WEEK: DAYS 8–15

Now that you have completed the store-cupboard cleanse, it is time to move to the next stage. Real Food Week is the first step towards a low-inflammatory keto diet, setting you up for health and longevity.

Your fridge should be brimming with fresh veggies – all different types of leaves and plenty of colour. Make veggies the hero by simply adding some fat, lemon, spices and/or sea salt. Real food contains more healthful 'information' that will nourish us. Perhaps reassess which ingredients are the hero on your plate. If protein has been the hero for years, please consider veggies to be the hero, with the protein being the 'condiment'.

Real Food Week is a celebration of veggies!

Aim to get your nutrients from the widest source possible. This might mean cooking with ingredients that haven't been on the radar before – so please try to be open-minded about that.

Please pay particular attention to your sleep during this week and beyond. The quantity as well as the quality of your sleep will affect the success of this protocol and moreover your health and longevity. See pages 115–16 for tips on optimising sleep.

From now on I am suggesting seven-day meal plans designed to be a guide, so feel free to select your own meals based on preferences.

	Breakfast	*Lunch*	*Dinner*
MONDAY	Kale and Chilli Omelette PAGE 153	Veggie Frittata PAGE 169	Baked Salmon in a Bag PAGE 197
TUESDAY	Baked Green Eggs PAGE 150	Roasted Veggies with Tahini Dressing PAGE 243	Beef Goulash PAGE 202
WEDNESDAY	Nutty Choc Smoothie PAGE 266	Quick and Easy Lamb PAGE 225	Pork Belly with Braised Cabbage PAGE 219
THURSDAY	Chia Pudding 1 PAGE 161 or Chia Pudding 2 PAGE 162	Salmon Parcels with a Mediterranean Medley PAGE 176	Bolognese PAGE 185
FRIDAY	Green Goddess PAGE 258	Veggie Medley PAGE 235	Coconut and Pumpkin Laksa PAGE 172
SATURDAY	Pesto Eggs PAGE 160	Snapper Stew PAGE 215	Vegetarian Korma PAGE 224
SUNDAY	Shakshuka PAGE 156	Asparagus Soup PAGE 174	Whole Baked Fish PAGE 226
Snacks	roasted macadamias, pâté, broth gummies		

TRANSITIONING 1: DAYS **16–23**

I'm allowing two weeks for this transitioning phase — some of us may take a little longer to adjust, so allow more time if necessary. If you are training at a high intensity, then you may need to dial this back for a few weeks as you transition and your body up-regulates the necessary pathways, *or* consider cyclic keto (see page 132).

Extending beyond the Real Food Week — this week we will start to manipulate your macronutrients to suit a higher fat protocol. We can begin to introduce some MCT to your diet to begin to elevate blood ketone levels. If you're new to MCT start with 1 teaspoon either straight off a spoon or in a smoothie.

Remember you will most likely feel like crap as you transition to a fat-burner — this is totally normal. At this point, having a buddy is pivotal! If you don't have a buddy, don't fear — simply use a friend as a sounding board and/or record your feelings in your journal.

Increase your water consumption — as your intake of fat increases and carbs decline, your natural ability to retain hydration is reduced, therefore ensure you're drinking appropriate amounts of water (0.04 × body mass kg = litres per day).

Start to foster an improved gut microbiome. The foods you're ingesting will naturally cultivate a healthier microbiome but you can introduce additional probiotics such as supplements, fermented foods, kombucha etc. Also, if you habitually sanitise every inch of your living space, maybe peel back on this a little.

	Breakfast	*Lunch*	*Dinner*
MONDAY	Baked Green Eggs PAGE 150	Pumpkin Frittata PAGE 165	Mexican Chicken and Easy Guacamole PAGE 186
TUESDAY	Kick Start PAGE 259	Pumpkin Soup with Crispy Bacon PAGE 173	Chilli Con Carne with Avo and Toms PAGE 221
WEDNESDAY	Sautéed Kale PAGE 234	Chicken Tacos with Guacamole PAGE 182	Pan-fried Snapper PAGE 188
THURSDAY	High-octane Coffee PAGE 253	Crispy-skin Sea Trout PAGE 191	Tandoori Chicken PAGE 209
FRIDAY	Buttery Scrambled Eggs and Bacon PAGE 157	Chicken Patties PAGE 168	Mussels in a Coconut Broth PAGE 208
SATURDAY	All the Greens PAGE 242	Jerk Chicken PAGE 212	Beef Stroganoff PAGE 213
SUNDAY	Bacon and Courgette Fritters PAGE 167	Asian Fish Cakes with Salad PAGE 170	Beef Rendang PAGE 207
Snacks	roasted macadamias, pâté, broth gummies		

TRANSITIONING 2: DAYS 24–31

If you've been diligent about your food, then you should be feeling a little more human during this second week of transitioning. It's fairly safe to say you won't have become fully fat-adapted, but you're well on your way. Training may still feel harder than usual, so just dial back the intensity or look at cyclic keto (see page 132).

Increase your intake of MCT oil to 1 tablespoon daily — either off the spoon or in your smoothie.

Incorporate some alternative ingredients and begin to be more adventurous with fat. Cooking with different types of fat (butter, ghee, beef dripping, duck fat, lard, coconut oil) will change the nuance of a dish.

How's the meditation going? Try to increase the duration of the meditation, but the important thing is consistency. There are plenty of apps you can download that will deliver guided meditation or similarly download binaural beats. Binaural beats help to induce a meditative state by manipulating the brain's frequency.

	Breakfast	*Lunch*	*Dinner*
MONDAY	Buttery Omelette PAGE 154	Pan-fried Hake PAGE 200	Moroccan Beef Stew PAGE 211
TUESDAY	The Fat Bomb PAGE 256	Poached Chicken in Broth PAGE 195	Whole Baked Snapper with Salsa Verde PAGE 201
WEDNESDAY	Powerhouse Smoothie PAGE 255	Grilled Mexican Chicken PAGE 196	Hoki in Coconut Broth PAGE 199
THURSDAY	Bulletproof Matcha Green Tea PAGE 264	Fuss-free Lamb Mince PAGE 229	Chicken One-pot PAGE 227
FRIDAY	The Anti-inflammatory Juice PAGE 267	Chicken Soup PAGE 164	Sausage Casserole PAGE 183
SATURDAY	Matcha Minty PAGE 261	Baked Brussels Sprouts with Tahini PAGE 233	Beef Cheeks in Chinese Five-spice PAGE 216
SUNDAY	Black Pudding and Eggs PAGE 149	Salmon Poke Bowl PAGE 166	Mexican Chicken and Easy Guacamole PAGE 186

Snacks   roasted macadamias, pâté, broth gummies

Now you're beyond the transitional phase . . . this is the good stuff — you have now engineered a diet that promotes the propagation of ketones in your liver which are available for energy for the entire body. Make sure you check in with your journal and in particular your mental clarity, mood and cognitive function. By now you should have ironed out the creases and should not be experiencing fluctuations in energy throughout the day. Remember the foods chosen in this 60-day protocol won't adversely affect your blood glucose/insulin, therefore facilitating consistent energy throughout the day.

A reminder that we should be getting our daily nutrients from varied sources. Try to introduce two or three new ingredients to the diet this week. Have you tried Jerusalem artichoke, bulletproof coffee, turmeric and/or mackerel?

If you haven't yet, I'd like you to introduce a fast. If you've never fasted before, don't panic — it's super-easy to integrate and be reassured your world won't cave in. If you attempted to fast on a high-carb diet, it would feel very different to how it will now at this stage of the protocol. Piggy-back on the fast we all naturally have during sleep and extend the gap between dinner the night before and breakfast the following morning. Aim for 16-plus hours, and when you end your fast do so with a fat-rich meal.

	Breakfast	*Lunch*	*Dinner*
MONDAY	Bulletproof Matcha Green Tea PAGE 264	Barbecue Prawns PAGE 228	Butter Chicken PAGE 203
TUESDAY (fast day)	Beef Bone Broth PAGE 246	Slow-cooked Lamb Shoulder with Roasted Veggies PAGE 178	Slow-cooked Osso Bucco PAGE 184
WEDNESDAY	Buttery Eggs with Salsa Verde and Heirloom Tomatoes PAGE 151	Liver and Onions PAGE 230	Poached Salmon with Courgette Ribbons PAGE 194
THURSDAY	Beef Bone Broth PAGE 246	Crispy-skin Sea Trout PAGE 191	Butter Chicken PAGE 203
FRIDAY	Leeks with Eggs and Salsa Verde PAGE 177	Veggie Medley PAGE 235	Roast Chicken with Baked Veggies PAGE 180
SATURDAY	Nearly Spanish Omelette PAGE 159	Pan-fried Sardines PAGE 175	Lamb and Bacon Casserole PAGE 204
SUNDAY	Black Pudding and Eggs PAGE 149	Baked Brussels Sprouts with Tahini PAGE 233	Irish Beef Stew PAGE 210
Snacks	roasted macadamias, pâté, broth gummies		

I'm incredibly excited for you at this stage — you're now 40 days in to a new approach to health and nutrition. You're laying down new habits and pathways ALL the time. You have been getting 80 per cent of your health from nutrition, so now it's time to take it to the next level and see what the remaining 20 per cent looks and feels like.

If you haven't considered exercise at this stage, then now is a great time. Before starting an exercise programme, be sure to get medical screening and a green light from your health practitioner. Embark on a programme that follows sequential development and enlist the help of an exercise professional. If cost is prohibitive, consider joining together with some friends/colleagues to reduce the cost per person.

NOOTROPIC FACTORS

Now is the time to optimise your cognitive function. Your brain has already being given high octane fuel through ketones but now let's 'optimise' this further. Begin to introduce some nootropics such as:

Turmeric — can be taken as a supplement or as a whole food. Turmeric will promote BDNF (brain-derived neurotrophic factors) — it's like a fertiliser for growth and repair of neurons.

Mushrooms — I could talk about mushrooms all day but I'll save you from that — instead I'll share what I consider the royalty of mushrooms:

King
chaga

Queen
reishi

Prince
cordyceps

Princess
lion's mane

These mushrooms, in particular, have powerful nootropic and 'adaptogen' properties — meaning they give us improved cognitive function and improved ability to cope with physiological stress. More and more products using these mushrooms are coming onto the market — keep an eye out for them and get into it!

	Breakfast	*Lunch*	*Dinner*
MONDAY (fast day)	High-octane Coffee PAGE 253 or Bulletproof Matcha Green Tea PAGE 264	Pumpkin Soup with Crispy Bacon PAGE 173	Whole Baked Fish PAGE 226
TUESDAY	Shakshuka PAGE 156	Pan-fried Hake PAGE 200	Beef Madras PAGE 214
WEDNESDAY (fast day)	Beef Bone Broth PAGE 246	Chicken Soup PAGE 164	Beef Cheeks in Chinese Five-spice PAGE 216
THURSDAY	All the Greens PAGE 242	Grilled Mexican Chicken PAGE 196	Meatballs in Tomato Sauce with Baked Pumpkin PAGE 189
FRIDAY	Choc Delight PAGE 254	Poached Chicken in Broth PAGE 195	Naked Burgers PAGE 192
SATURDAY	Buttery Scrambled Eggs and Bacon PAGE 157	Mushrooms in Butter and Thyme PAGE 240	Coconut and Pumpkin Laksa PAGE 172
SUNDAY	Nearly Spanish Omelette PAGE 159	Chicken Tacos with Guacamole PAGE 182	Bolognese PAGE 185

Snacks   roasted macadamias, pâté, broth, gummies

Fun fact — the largest single living organism on the planet is found in a forest in Oregon. It's found beneath the surface and is the tendrils or network of mushrooms. The mycelium is the 'mother' or network for the flowering mushroom above ground — google mycelium and prepare to be mind-blown!

Introduce an additional fast — incorporate two fasts in your week, aiming for at least 16 hours each.

OFF-RAMP: DAYS 50-60

You now have all the information to make informed choices around nutrition, supplementation and bio-hacking. This is the final week of the 60-day protocol and a time to metaphorically detach — and to be in the driver's seat for your health. If in doubt, ask yourself is this food or practice going to induce inflammation that will be detrimental to my health in the long term?

Continue to implement supplementation and strategies to enhance your health and optimise cognitive function. See Chapter Eight for information on nootropics and supplementation.

Try infra-red sauna or traditional sauna (obtain the green light from your health practitioner first) as a great way to boost immunity.

Mindfulness — continue to meditate as consistently as you can.

During this final week I'd love for you to integrate a longer fast — aim for 18–24 hours (again, obtain a green light from your health practitioner beforehand) and include one of these longer fasts once or twice a year.

At the end of this final week, I'd like you to reflect on your progress. Refer back to your journal and the early entries — compare and contrast how you feel. Analyse every aspect of your health and how it's changed over time.

Do you have increased energy levels? Improved mood? Have you lost body fat? Reduced brain fog? Have the aches and pains diminished? Does food energise you now?

	Breakfast	*Lunch*	*Dinner*
MONDAY (fast day)	High-octane Coffee PAGE 253	Butter Chicken PAGE 203	
TUESDAY	Pesto Eggs PAGE 160	Snapper Stew PAGE 215	Pork Belly with Braised Cabbage PAGE 219
WEDNESDAY	All the Greens PAGE 242	Grilled Mexican Chicken PAGE 196	Poached Salmon with Courgette Ribbons PAGE 194
THURSDAY (fast day)	The Anti-inflammatory Juice PAGE 267	Roasted Bone Marrow with Chimichurri PAGE 231	Lamb Shank Ragu with Cauli 'n' Broccoli Rice PAGE 217
FRIDAY	Kale and Chilli Omelette PAGE 153	Mushrooms in Butter and Thyme PAGE 240	Vegetarian Korma PAGE 224
SATURDAY	Gut-healing Smoothie PAGE 260	Fuss-free Lamb Mince PAGE 229	Mussels in a Coconut Broth PAGE 208
SUNDAY	Black Pudding and Eggs PAGE 149	Chicken Tacos with Guacamole PAGE 182	Whole Baked Fish PAGE 226
Snacks	roasted macadamias, pâté, broth gummies		

If you have been disciplined with the 60-day protocol, congratulations are in order! You should have seen marked improvements across many facets of your health. I strongly advise you to continue with your journey, making your own body and brain a case study for further optimisation!

A note on ingredients: The quality of energy you get out of your body is only as good as the quality you put into it, so always try to use the best ingredients you can if they're affordable. Where possible, choose biodynamic/organic free-range eggs and chicken, grass-fed meat and organic fruit and veggies. Also, use good-quality oils and sea salt and freshly ground black pepper.

BREAKFAST

Black Pudding and Eggs

If I had to choose my last supper before meeting my end, it would almost certainly include black pudding or black sausage. Look beyond what black sausage actually is and judge it only for its texture and flavour – which is hard to beat!

SERVES 4

300 g gluten-free black pudding, sliced into 1 cm discs
6 eggs
1 tablespoon butter
sea salt and freshly ground black pepper, to taste

1. Heat a frying pan over medium–high heat and add the sausage. Cook for 3–4 minutes on each side, or until crispy on the outside and cooked through. Remove from the pan and set aside.
2. Crack the eggs into a bowl and use a fork to lightly whisk.
3. Return the pan to the hob over low heat. Add the butter, then add the whisked eggs and cook for 4–5 minutes, gently folding with a spatula until cooked to your liking. Remove from the heat, season with salt and pepper, and serve with the black sausage.

Baked Green Eggs

Nothing is more seductive than lashings of butter, and when combined with leeks it's a match made in heaven. If you like you can add a little Salsa Verde (see recipe page 151) to provide acidity and cut through the richness of this dish.

SERVES 1-2

2 tablespoons butter
1 long red chilli, *deseeded and chopped*
handful of Brussels sprouts, *trimmed and halved*
½ leek, *chopped*
2–4 eggs
handful of parsley, *chopped*
sea salt and freshly ground black pepper, to taste

1. Place a frying pan over low heat, add the butter, then add the chilli and Brussels sprouts and cook for 1 minute. Add the leek and cook for 5–6 minutes, stirring occasionally.
2. Make depressions in the veggies and crack the eggs in. Cook for a further 5–6 minutes, or until the eggs are cooked to your liking.
3. Remove from the heat, add the parsley, and season with salt and pepper. Serve with salsa verde on the side.

Buttery Eggs with Salsa Verde and Heirloom Tomatoes

Eggs for breakfast are nothing new, so I'm always trying to mix in elements that brighten them up. Here the salsa verde cuts through the buttery eggs and is an absolute winner!

SERVES 2-4

3 heirloom tomatoes, *halved*
1 tablespoon olive oil
sea salt and freshly ground black pepper, to taste
4-6 eggs
1 tablespoon butter

SALSA VERDE

large handful of parsley
½ handful of basil
¼ handful of mint
4 tablespoons olive oil
splash of apple cider vinegar
1 tablespoon lemon juice
1 garlic clove roughly chopped
3 anchovies (optional)
3 cornichons (baby pickled cucumbers)
freshly ground black pepper, to taste

1. Preheat your oven to 180°C.
2. Place the halved tomatoes on a baking tray lined with baking paper. Dress with olive oil, season with salt and pepper and bake for 15–20 minutes, or until softened. When cooked, remove from the oven.
3. Meanwhile, whiz all the ingredients for the salsa verde in a blender until just combined.
4. Lightly whisk the eggs in a bowl.
5. Place a frying pan over low–medium heat, add the butter, then add the eggs and cook for 5–6 minutes, or until cooked to your liking (for best results cook low and long). Remove from the heat.
6. Serve the eggs with the baked tomatoes and a drizzle of the salsa verde.

Kale and Chilli Omelette

SERVES 1

1 tablespoon butter, ghee or coconut oil
½ brown onion, *finely chopped*
1 long red chilli, *deseeded and roughly chopped*
¼ bunch of kale, *trimmed and roughly chopped*
4 eggs
sea salt and freshly ground black pepper, to taste

1. Place a frying pan over medium heat, add the fat, then add the onion and chilli. Cook, stirring, until the onion begins to soften. Remove from the pan and set aside.

2. Add some more fat to the pan if necessary and throw in the chopped kale. Toss gently until the kale begins to wilt and soften, then remove and set aside with the onion mixture.

3. Lightly beat the eggs in a bowl. Return the pan to the hob over medium heat and pour the egg into the pan. After 30 seconds, cover half the omelette with the onion, chilli and kale. Cook for 2 minutes, or until you can lift the egg with a spatula without it losing shape. Lift the omelette opposite the kale mixture and flip it over to cover, then continue to cook for 2–3 minutes, or until cooked to your liking.

4. Remove from the heat, season with salt and pepper, and serve.

Buttery Omelette

SERVES 1

4 eggs
2 tablespoons butter
1 small brown onion, *sliced*
sea salt and freshly ground black pepper, to taste

1. Lightly beat the eggs in a bowl.
2. Place a frying pan over low heat, add the butter, then add the onion and sauté for 3–4 minutes, or until softened. Spread the onion evenly around the pan, then pour in the eggs and cook for 3–4 minutes, or until the underside is cooked and the edges are firm.
3. Using a spatula, lift the edge and fold one side across to the other to close the omelette. At this stage you can either throw it in a preheated 180°C oven for 4–5 minutes or continue to cook on the hob for 4–5 minutes.
4. Remove from the heat, season with salt and pepper, and serve.

Eggs with Extras

SERVES **2**

3 tablespoons butter
4 shallots, *finely chopped*
2 garlic cloves, *finely chopped*
1 long red chilli, *finely chopped*
½ bunch of kale, *trimmed and chopped*
4 eggs
sea salt and freshly ground black pepper, to taste

1. Place a frying pan over medium heat, add the butter, then add the shallots, garlic and chilli. Cook for 3–4 minutes, or until softened, then add the kale. Stir to combine, then cook for a further 1 minute.
2. Make four hollows in the kale mix and crack an egg into each. Cook for 4–5 minutes, or until the eggs are cooked to your liking. Season with salt and pepper, and serve.

Shakshuka

SERVES 2

2 tablespoons butter or olive oil
1 brown onion, *chopped*
2 garlic cloves, *chopped*
2 × 400 g tins diced tomatoes
1 red pepper, *deseeded and chopped*
1 teaspoon cumin
½ teaspoon cayenne pepper
1 teaspoon paprika
handful of parsley, *chopped*
4 eggs
sea salt and freshly ground black pepper, to taste

1. Heat a frying pan over medium heat, add the butter or oil, then add the onion and garlic and cook for 3–4 minutes, or until softened.

2. Add the tomato, peppers and spices and cook for a further 3–4 minutes. Stir in the parsley.

3. Make four hollows in the tomato mixture and crack an egg into each. Cook for 4–5 minutes, or until the eggs are cooked to your liking. Season with salt and pepper, and serve.

Buttery Scrambled Eggs and Bacon

SERVES **2**

4 eggs
2 tablespoons butter
4 rashers of bacon
sea salt and freshly ground black pepper, to taste

1. In a mixing bowl, gently whisk the eggs and butter. Set aside.
2. Place a frying pan over high heat, add the bacon and cook for 2–3 minutes on each side, or until cooked to your liking. Remove from the pan and set aside.
3. Return the pan to the hob and turn the heat off. Remove excess fat if you wish, but leave some for flavour. Pour the egg mixture into the pan – there should be enough residual heat to slowly cook the eggs. Once cooked to your liking, remove from the heat, season with salt and pepper, and serve.

Baked Eggs with Buttery Leeks

SERVES **2**

2 tablespoons butter
1 leek, *sliced*
1 long red chilli, *deseeded and finely chopped*
large handful of Brussels sprouts, *trimmed and sliced*
4 eggs
sea salt and freshly ground black pepper, to taste
2 tablespoons Salsa Verde (see recipe page 151)

1. Place a frying pan over medium heat, add the butter, then add the leek, chilli and Brussels sprouts. Sauté for 4–5 minutes, or until the veggies begin to soften.
2. Make four hollows in the mixture and crack an egg into each.
3. Cook over low–medium heat for 4–5 minutes, or until the eggs are cooked to your liking. Remove from the heat, season with salt and pepper, and drizzle with the salsa verde. Serve.

Nearly Spanish Omelette

This is a 'nearly' Spanish omelette because it does away with potato. It's a simple recipe and should be in your repertoire for those times you have guests over for breakfast. The sweet sautéed onion is the hero of the dish, but if you don't have 25 minutes to caramelise your onion, simply sauté it for 3–4 minutes on a slightly higher heat, just until it turns translucent.

SERVES 2

6–8 eggs
1 tablespoon butter
1 tablespoon olive oil
1 red onion, *finely sliced*
1 long red chilli (optional), *deseeded and finely chopped*
¼ bunch of fresh parsley, *roughly chopped*
sea salt and freshly ground black pepper, to taste

1. Preheat your oven to 180°C.
2. In a bowl, lightly whisk the eggs.
3. Place a frying pan over low heat and add the butter and olive oil. Add the onion and cook for 25–30 minutes, or until caramelised. Add the chilli towards the end of the caramelisation process and 5 minutes before adding the eggs.
4. Keeping the pan over low heat, add the eggs. Top with the parsley, season with salt and pepper, and cook for 3–4 minutes, or until the base is lightly browned. Lift one side and fold over to the opposite, effectively halving the omelette. Transfer to the oven and bake for 5–6 minutes, or until cooked to your liking. Remove from the heat and season again, if desired.

Pesto Eggs

SERVES **2**

6–8 eggs
1 tablespoon butter
1–2 tablespoons Pesto (see recipe page 250)
sea salt and freshly ground black pepper, to taste

1. In a bowl, lightly whisk the eggs.
2. Place a frying pan over low heat and add the butter. Pour in the egg and stir occasionally with a wooden spoon or spatula for 4–5 minutes, or until cooked to your liking. (Remember, the egg will continue to cook once removed from the pan due to residual heat, so err on the side of undercooking it.) Stir the pesto through and season with salt and pepper.

Chia Pudding 1

Easy to prepare the night before for a quick, fuss-free start to the day!

SERVES 2

¼ cup chia seeds
1 cup coconut milk or nut milk
1 teaspoon cinnamon
1 teaspoon vanilla extract
½–1 teaspoon honey (optional)
crushed berries, to top
toasted coconut, to top

1. Combine all the ingredients, with the exception of the berries and toasted coconut, in a mixing bowl. Spoon the mixture into serving glasses and place in the refrigerator for at least 1 hour or preferably overnight. To serve, top with berries and coconut, or anything crunchy to your liking.

Chia Pudding 2

SERVES **2**

¼ cup chia seeds
400 ml coconut cream
1 teaspoon vanilla extract
½ teaspoon cinnamon
¼ teaspoon nutmeg
1 teaspoon honey (optional)
splash of water
handful of crushed nuts or shredded coconut

1. Combine all the ingredients except the nuts/coconut in a mixing
   bowl. Leave to stand for 15 minutes, then cover and pop into the
   fridge until morning. To serve, top with crushed nuts or shredded
   coconut.

LUNCH

Grilled Mackerel

SERVES 2

2 small whole mackerel, gutted and cleaned
2 tablespoons olive oil
1 long red chilli, *deseeded and finely chopped*
sea salt and freshly ground black pepper, to taste
juice of 1 lemon
¼ bunch of coriander, *roughly chopped*

1. Preheat the oven to 180°C.
2. Place the mackerel on a baking tray lined with baking paper. Drizzle with oil, sprinkle with chilli, and season with salt and pepper. Bake in the oven for 12–15 minutes, or until cooked to your liking. (Cooking time will vary depending on the size of the fish.)
3. Remove from the oven and allow the fish to rest a few moments, then squeeze over the lemon, sprinkle with coriander and serve.

Chicken Soup

Chicken soup is the go-to dish for nursing a loved one back to health after an illness. Its health benefits may seem like an old wives' tale, but the bones/joints actually do offer therapeutic properties. You can add a chicken carcass to this recipe, if you wish. Once you add the broth, throw in a carcass, and remove it before the end.

SERVES 4

2 tablespoons olive oil or butter
1 onion, *chopped*
3 garlic cloves, *chopped*
2 celery sticks, *chopped*
2 carrots, *chopped*
1 bay leaf
2 sprigs of thyme
2 litres Chicken Bone Broth (see recipe page 247)
½ pumpkin (about 400 g), *cut into 2 cm chunks*
400 g shredded cooked chicken
1 handful of peas (frozen is fine)
sea salt and freshly ground black pepper, to taste
juice of ½ lemon
¼ bunch of parsley, *roughly chopped*

1. Place a large saucepan over medium heat, add the oil or butter, then add the onion, garlic, celery, carrot, bay leaf and thyme. Cook, stirring occasionally, for 5–6 minutes, or until the onion has softened. Add the broth and bring to the boil, then reduce the heat and simmer for 15 minutes.
2. Add the pumpkin and cook for a further 15 minutes, or until softened. Add the chicken and peas and cook for 5–6 minutes.
3. Remove from the heat, season with salt and pepper, and add the lemon juice. Serve into bowls and sprinkle with parsley.

Pumpkin Frittata

Having a yummy frittata recipe up your sleeve is a must. This recipe is perfect to keep the kids happy at dinnertime but can double up nicely as a breakfast item. Feel free to add some bacon. Simply crisp up 4 rashers in a frying pan and, once the fat is rendered, remove from the heat and chop. Add to the mixture before putting it in the oven.

SERVES 4

340 g chopped pumpkin
½ teaspoon sea salt
2 tablespoons olive oil
1 tablespoon butter, plus extra for greasing
1 brown onion, *sliced*
½ leek, *sliced*
1 bunch of asparagus, *trimmed and chopped*
sea salt and freshly ground black pepper, to taste
1 tablespoon finely chopped chives
10 eggs

1. Preheat your oven to 180°C. Place the pumpkin pieces on a lined baking tray, season with the sea salt, drizzle with the olive oil and roast for 35 minutes.
2. Meanwhile, grease a 20 cm × 30 cm baking dish with a little butter.
3. Place a frying pan over low heat, add the remaining butter, then add the onion, leek and asparagus and cook for 4–5 minutes, or until the vegetables are just softened. Remove from the heat, add salt and pepper to taste, then stir in the chives.
4. In a bowl, lightly whisk the eggs.
5. Transfer the veggie mixture into your prepared baking dish, add the baked pumpkin and pour the egg over the top. Place in the oven. Cook for 40 minutes, or until lightly browned and cooked through. Serve warm.

Salmon Poke Bowl

SERVES 1

DRESSING

1 garlic clove, *finely chopped*
1 cm knob of root ginger, *peeled and finely chopped*
1 long red chilli, *finely chopped*
juice of 2 limes
1 teaspoon fish sauce (nam pla)
½ teaspoon honey

POKE BOWL

1 salmon fillet
½ avocado, *sliced*
1 carrot, *chopped or coarsely grated*
½ cucumber, *diced*
¼ red cabbage, *finely chopped*
¼ bunch of coriander, *roughly chopped*
1 long red or green chilli, *finely chopped*
handful of salad leaves
1 shallot, *finely chopped*
1 tablespoon sesame seeds, to serve

1. Combine all the ingredients for the dressing in a small bowl and whisk together. Set aside to allow the flavours to infuse.
2. Bring some salted water to the boil in a saucepan, place the salmon fillet in the water and turn off the heat. Allow the salmon to sit in the water for 8–10 minutes, depending on the size of the fillet. Remove from the water and pull the fillet into flakes.
3. Arrange the remaining salad ingredients in the bowl, top with the salmon pieces, sprinkle with sesame seeds and drizzle with the dressing.

Bacon and Courgette Fritters

MAKES 12 FRITTERS

2 rashers of bacon
2 courgettes, *seeds removed, grated*
1 carrot, *grated*
1 shallot, *finely chopped*
2 eggs
2 tablespoons ground almonds
1 teaspoon cumin
1 teaspoon turmeric
¼ teaspoon baking powder
1 tablespoon butter or ghee
sea salt and freshly ground black pepper, to taste

1. Place a large frying pan over high heat, add the bacon and cook for 2–3 minutes on each side, or until crispy. Remove from the pan and set aside.
2. In a mixing bowl, combine all the remaining ingredients except the butter or ghee. chop the cooked bacon into small pieces and add to the mixture. Combine well.
3. Return the frying pan to a medium heat and add the butter or ghee. Drop 2 heaped tablespoons of batter onto the pan per fritter. Cook fritters for around 3 minutes on each side before removing from the heat. Keep fritters warm prior to serving.

Chicken Patties

SERVES **4**

500 g chicken mince
1 long red chilli, *chopped*
1 garlic clove, *finely chopped*
¼ bunch of coriander, *roughly chopped*
¼ bunch of mint, *roughly chopped*
1 teaspoon cumin
1 teaspoon paprika
1 egg yolk
sea salt and freshly ground black pepper, to taste
1 tablespoon butter or coconut oil

1. In a large mixing bowl, combine the chicken mince, chilli, garlic, fresh herbs, spices and egg. Season with salt and pepper and mix well.
2. Place a frying pan over medium heat and add the butter or coconut oil. Divide the chicken mix into four even-sized patties. Place them into the pan and cook for 4–5 minutes on each side, or until cooked through. Remove from the heat and serve.

Veggie Frittata

SERVES 4

1 tablespoon butter or coconut oil, plus extra for greasing
1 onion, *chopped*
2 garlic cloves, *chopped*
200 g cherry tomatoes, *halved*
handful of kale leaves, *chopped*
1 kg courgettes, *grated and squeezed of excess moisture*
6 eggs
¼ bunch of flat-leaf parsley, *chopped*
sea salt and freshly ground black pepper, to taste

1. Preheat your oven to 190°C. Grease a 20 cm × 30 cm baking dish with oil.
2. Place a large frying pan over low heat, add the butter or coconut oil, then add the onion and garlic and sauté for 3–4 minutes. Add the tomatoes, kale and courgettes and cook for 8–10 minutes, or until most of the moisture has been removed. Remove from the heat and set aside.
3. In a large mixing bowl, gently whisk the eggs and stir in the parsley. Add the veggie mixture and season with salt and pepper.
4. Pour the frittata mixture into the prepared baking dish. Place in the oven and cook for 40 minutes, or until cooked through and browned on top. Remove from the heat. Add extra seasonings, if desired, and serve warm.

Asian Fish Cakes with Salad

The flavours in these fish cakes will remind you of Thai holidays. It'll work with most fish.

SERVES 2-4

2 medium fish fillets (e.g. trout, salmon, hake, John Dory), *skin off*
½ red onion, *finely chopped*
½ bunch of coriander, *stalks and leaves roughly chopped*
zest of 2 limes
3 eggs
2 garlic cloves, *crushed*
2 cm knob of root ginger, *peeled and crushed*
4 small red chillies
½ teaspoon sea salt
1–2 tablespoons coconut flour
1 tablespoon coconut oil

SALAD

handful of basil leaves
handful of mint leaves
2 shallots, *finely chopped*
macadamia or olive oil

1. Chop the fish fillets up into small chunks.
2. In a mixing bowl, combine the fish, onion, coriander, lime zest, eggs, garlic, ginger, chilli and salt. Mix well, gradually adding the coconut flour. The mixture should resemble a sticky dough and should hold together when compacted.
3. Place a frying pan over medium heat and add the coconut oil. Divide the mixture into 4–6 balls. Place the balls in the pan, pressing down with a spatula to form patties. Cook for 2–3 minutes on each side, depending on how thick your patties are. Remove and keep warm while you combine the basil, mint and shallots. Dress lightly with macadamia or olive oil and serve the salad alongside the fish cakes.

Coconut and Pumpkin Laksa

This recipe is super-comforting, with plenty of 'information'-rich foods to promote health and longevity.

SERVES 4

2 tablespoons coconut oil
2 garlic cloves, *crushed*
3 teaspoons Thai seven-spice
2–3 cm knob of root ginger, *peeled and minced*
2 stalks of lemongrass, white part only, *thinly sliced*
1 bird's-eye chilli, *finely chopped*
300 g butternut squash, *chopped*
300 g cauliflower, *cut into small florets*
1 red pepper, *deseeded and chopped*
1 green pepper, *deseeded and chopped*
1 × 400 ml tin coconut cream
200 ml vegetable broth
1 teaspoon tamarind paste
100 g baby spinach
¼ bunch of coriander leaves

1. Place a large saucepan over medium heat, add the coconut oil, then add the garlic, Thai seven-spice, ginger, lemongrass and chilli and cook for 4–5 minutes. Add the butternut squash and cauliflower and toss through. Cook for 2–3 minutes before adding the red and green peppers, coconut cream and broth.
2. Cook for several minutes, or until the squash is cooked through and sauce is thickened to your liking. Add the tamarind paste and spinach and stir through. Once the spinach has softened (1–2 minutes), remove from the heat. Add the coriander leaves and stir through before serving.

Pumpkin Soup with Crispy Bacon

Warm and comforting, this is a soup to soothe your soul.

SERVES 4

2 tablespoons olive oil
1 large brown onion, *chopped*
4 garlic cloves, *chopped*
2 celery sticks, *sliced*
2 carrots, *sliced*
2 bay leaves
1 sprig of thyme
1 teaspoon chopped fresh or dried sage
2 litres Chicken Bone Broth (see recipe page 247) or Vegetable
  Broth
750 g pumpkin, *roughly chopped*
250 g streaky bacon
200 ml coconut cream (optional)
sea salt and freshly ground black pepper, to taste
½ bunch of parsley, *roughly chopped*

1. Place a large saucepan over low–medium heat and add the oil. Add
   the onion, garlic, celery, carrot and herbs and sauté for 5–6 minutes,
   stirring occasionally. Pour in the broth and cook for a further 10
   minutes, then add the pumpkin and allow to simmer for 10–15 minutes,
   or until the pumpkin begins to soften. Remove from the heat, allow
   to cool a little, then blitz in a food processor or blender – you may
   need to do this in batches. Return to the saucepan over low heat.
2. Meanwhile, place a frying pan over medium–high heat and add the
   bacon. Cook for 2–3 minutes on each side, or until crispy. Remove
   from the heat and set aside. Once cooled, roughly chop.
3. Remove the soup from the heat, add the coconut cream, if using,
   and season to taste with salt and pepper. Stir through the parsley
   and bacon, and serve.

Asparagus Soup

Rather than only using the sweet tips of the asparagus, this recipe will include a good part of the stalks, which increases the resistant starch content to feed our gut microbes.

SERVES 4

1 kg asparagus
2 tablespoons butter
1 brown onion, *roughly chopped*
1 litre Vegetable Broth (see recipe page 248) or Chicken Bone Broth (see recipe page 247)
small handful of basil leaves, *roughly chopped*
sea salt and freshly ground black pepper, to taste
200 ml coconut cream

1. Discard the very ends of your asparagus stalks and roughly chop the rest.
2. Place a large saucepan over low–medium heat and add the butter, then add the onion and sauté for 3–4 minutes, or until softened. Add the asparagus and cook for a further 2–3 minutes. Add the broth and basil, and season with salt and pepper. Bring to the boil, then reduce to a simmer and cook for 30 minutes.
3. Remove from the heat, allow to cool a little, then blitz in a food processor or blender – you may need to do this in batches. Return to the saucepan over low heat. Stir in the coconut cream, adjust seasonings if required, and serve.

Pan-fried Sardines

Sardines tick a few boxes. Firstly, they are one of the more affordable fish at the fishmonger's. Secondly, being lower down the food chain they are less affected by the heavy metal accumulation associated with bigger predatory fish such as tuna and salmon. Lastly, they are a rich source of EPA and DHA, important fatty acids.

SERVES 4

2 tablespoons olive oil
1 long green chilli, *deseeded and roughly chopped*
2 garlic cloves, *roughly chopped*
24 fresh sardines, *gutted and cleaned*
juice and zest of 1 lemon
¼ bunch of parsley, *roughly chopped*
sea salt and freshly ground black pepper, to taste

1. Place a large frying pan over medium heat, add the oil, then add the chilli and garlic and cook for 30 seconds. Add the sardines and cook for 1–2 minutes on each side. You may have to cook these in batches.
2. Remove from the heat and transfer to a large plate. Top with the lemon juice, lemon zest and parsley, and season with salt and pepper. Serve immediately.

Salmon Parcels with a Mediterranean Medley

I love this recipe. Last summer I discovered it to be quite the crowd pleaser for picnics. Simply chuck the parcels in the oven 8–10 minutes before heading out the door. In the time it takes to get you and your hamper to the park, the fish will have been allowed to rest for just the right length of time.

SERVES 2

¼ baby fennel, *cored and sliced*
200 g of cherry tomatoes, *halved*
60 g kalamata olives, *roughly chopped*
2 tablespoons olive oil
1 lemon, *sliced (3 slices per fillet)*
2 salmon fillets
2 sprigs of dill
sea salt and freshly ground black pepper, to taste

1. Preheat your oven to 180°C.
2. In a mixing bowl, combine the fennel, tomato and olives and drizzle with half of the olive oil.
3. Cut two large squares of baking paper. Place the sliced lemon in the middle of the paper sheets and place a salmon fillet on top. Top with the dill sprigs and pour the fennel mixture on and around the salmon. Drizzle with the remaining olive oil and season with salt and pepper.
4. Create a parcel by grabbing the four corners of the paper and bringing them together before tying with baking twine. Place on a baking tray and bake in the oven for 8–10 minutes, or until the fish is just cooked through. Allow to rest for 3–4 minutes before cutting the parcels open with scissors.

Leeks with Eggs and Salsa Verde

SERVES 1

1 tablespoon butter or olive oil
12 Brussels sprouts, *sliced or shredded*
¼ leek, *sliced*
2 eggs
sea salt and freshly ground black pepper, to taste
Salsa Verde (see recipe page 151)

1. Place a frying pan over medium heat and add the butter or oil. Add the Brussels sprouts and cook for 1 minute, then add the leeks. Reduce the heat to low and cook for 5–6 minutes, or until the veggies begin to soften.
2. Make two hollows in the vegetable mixture and crack the eggs into the depressions. Cook over low–medium heat for 4–5 minutes, or until eggs are cooked to your liking. Remove from the heat and season with salt and pepper. Serve with the salsa verde.

DINNER

Slow-cooked Lamb Shoulder with Roasted Veggies

I absolutely love slow-cooked recipes, and for good reasons. Firstly, they are fuss-free: I simply set and go, which allows me time to get on with my day. Secondly, the cuts of meat I use are typically more affordable and contain more of the 'good stuff', which is always a tick in my mind.

SERVES 4

1 shoulder of lamb, *bone in*
1 sprig of thyme
1 sprig of rosemary
6 brown onions, *peeled and quartered*
6 garlic cloves, *whole*
1 litre Beef Bone Broth (see recipe page 246)
450 g pumpkin, *sliced*
4 red onions, *peeled and halved*
3 heads of garlic, *halved crossways*
3 tablespoons olive oil
sea salt and freshly ground black pepper, to taste

1. Preheat your oven to 250°C.
2. Select a lidded ovenproof dish that is large enough to contain the lamb shoulder. Place the lamb in the dish, scatter over the herbs and surround with the onion and garlic. Pour enough broth into the dish to cover at least three-quarters of the lamb. Pop the lid on and place in the oven, immediately reducing the temperature to 140°C. Cook for 4 hours, or until the meat starts to fall off the bone. Remove from the heat and allow to rest, with the lid on.
3. Reset the oven temperature to 180°C. Line a baking tray with baking paper.
4. Place the pumpkin, red onion and garlic in a large mixing bowl, add the olive oil and season with salt and pepper. Stir well, then tip the veggies onto the baking tray and roast for 35–45 minutes, or until the veggies are softened and browned.
5. Just before the veggies are ready, pull the lamb meat away from the bone. Arrange on a platter with the baked veggies, and serve.

Roast Chicken with Baked Veggies

A roast chicken is hard to beat, if it's done well. This recipe delivers succulent chicken with a crispy skin every time. Cooking times will vary according to chicken size and efficiency of your oven. Note that beef dripping is used in this recipe. Dripping is the fat from beef and can be sourced from some butcher's. It will bring richness to the veggies, as will duck fat.

SERVES 4

1 whole chicken
½ brown onion, *peeled*
½ lemon
1 sprig of lemon thyme
1 tablespoon butter
2 tablespoons olive oil
sea salt and freshly ground black pepper, to taste
2 parsnips, *trimmed and halved*
4 heads of garlic, *halved crossways*
4 carrots, *cut into batons*
250 g pumpkin, *roughly chopped*
4 red onions, *peeled and quartered*
2 tablespoons beef dripping or olive oil
sea salt and freshly ground black pepper, to taste
2 sprigs of rosemary
2 sprigs of thyme

1. Preheat your oven to 250°C.
2. Begin by preparing the chicken. Insert the onion, lemon half and sprig of lemon thyme into the cavity of the chicken. Make a small incision beneath the skin and breast. Insert the butter under the skin.
3. Place the chicken in a roasting pan, drizzle with the olive oil and season with salt and pepper.
4. In a large mixing bowl, combine the veggies, drizzle with beef dripping or olive oil and season with salt and pepper. Line a baking tray with baking paper and spread the veggies over the baking tray. Scatter over the sprigs of rosemary and thyme.
5. Pop the chicken into the oven on the high shelf and reduce the temperature to 190°C. Place the veggies on the shelf below. Cook for 1 hour (depending on the size of the chicken).
6. Remove the chicken from the oven cover with foil and allow it to rest for 10 minutes. Season again with salt and pepper, if desired, and serve with the baked vegetables.

Chicken Tacos with Guacamole

A recipe that the kids will love, and perfect to use when you have leftover chicken. If you can't get hold of baby radicchio and cos lettuce, an iceberg lettuce will work.

SERVES 4

1 small red onion, *finely chopped*
3 ripe avocados
juice of 1–2 limes
¼ bunch of coriander (optional), *chopped*
sea salt and freshly ground black pepper, to taste
2 tomatoes, *seeds removed, diced*
8 baby radicchio leaves
8 baby cos lettuce leaves
500 g shredded cooked chicken

1. Pop the onion in a bowl and cover with water. Soak for 5–10 minutes, then rinse and drain.
2. To make the guacamole, remove the flesh from the avocados, place in a mixing bowl and mash with a fork. Add lime juice to taste. Add coriander, if using, and the chopped onion. Season with salt and pepper.
3. Place a teaspoonful of chopped tomato in each radicchio and cos lettuce leaf. Top with a small handful of shredded chicken and 1 tablespoon of guacamole. Season with more salt and pepper, if desired.

Sausage Casserole

There are no rules when it comes to which sausage to choose for this recipe – it'll help to select your kids' favourites. I'm a big fan of mushrooms, not just because of their taste and texture but because some mushrooms are amongst the most nutrient-dense foods on the planet. If your kids aren't lovers of mushrooms, feel free to leave them out of the recipe.

SERVES 4

2 tablespoons olive oil
¼ bunch of parsley, *stalks finely chopped and leaves roughly chopped*
2 onions, *chopped*
2 garlic cloves, *chopped*
6 large gluten-free sausages
1 litre Beef Bone Broth (see recipe page 246)
½ sprig of rosemary
½ butternut squash (about 500 g), *chopped*
2 carrots, *chopped*
handful of mushrooms (optional)
sea salt and freshly ground black pepper, to taste

1. Preheat your oven to 160°C.
2. Place the olive oil in a large frying pan over medium heat, add the parsley stalks, onion, garlic and sausages and cook until the sausages are golden. Remove from the heat and transfer to an ovenproof dish.
3. Add the broth, rosemary, squash and carrot and pop the casserole into the oven. Bake for 30 minutes, then remove and add the mushrooms. Gently combine. Bake for a further 20 minutes.
4. Remove from the oven, pour the liquid into a saucepan and rapidly reduce the liquid over high heat. Return the reduction to the dish, add the parsley leaves, season with salt and pepper, and serve.

Slow-cooked Osso Bucco

This was my late father's favourite, and a dish I always used to wonder about when he ordered it in restaurants . . . it sounded so intriguing! Osso bucco is a dish that uses veal shanks and requires long, slow cooking.

SERVES 4

2 tablespoons butter
4–6 veal shanks
2 brown onions, *chopped*
4 garlic cloves, *chopped*
4 carrots, *roughly chopped*
1 celery stalk, *roughly chopped*
2 teaspoons dried oregano
2 teaspoons dried thyme
1 bay leaf
400 g chopped tomatoes (fresh or tinned)
600 ml Beef Bone Broth (see recipe page 246),
sea salt and freshly ground black pepper, to taste

1. Preheat the oven to its highest temperature setting.
2. Place a large frying pan over medium–high heat and add 1 tablespoon of the butter. Add the meat and brown off, turning to ensure both sides are browned. Transfer to a lidded ovenproof dish.
3. Place the frying pan over low heat, add the remaining butter and sauté the onion and garlic for 3–4 minutes. Add the carrot, celery and herbs and stir for a further 3–4 minutes, coating the ingredients with the herbs. Add more butter if you need to. Remove from the heat and transfer to the ovenproof dish with the veal.
4. Add the tomato and beef broth and gently combine. Pop the lid on the casserole and put it in the oven. Immediately reduce the heat to 150°C and cook for 2½ hours, or until the meat starts to fall off the bone. Remove from the heat and season to taste.

Bolognese

SERVES 4

2 tablespoons olive oil
1 brown onion, *sliced*
3 garlic cloves, *chopped*
2 carrots, *diced*
1 celery stalk, *chopped*
1 sprig of thyme
2 teaspoons dried oregano
2 bay leaves
1 kg beef mince
800 g chopped tomatoes (fresh or tinned)
100 ml tomato passata
500 ml Beef Bone Broth (see recipe page 246)
4 large field mushrooms, *quartered*
500 g pumpkin, *roughly chopped*
sea salt and freshly ground black pepper, to taste

1. Place a heavy-based saucepan over medium heat, add the oil, then add the onion, garlic, carrot and celery and sauté for 4–5 minutes. Add the herbs, then turn the heat up and throw in the mince. Keep stirring until all the mince is browned. Throw in the chopped tomato, tomato passata and broth. Stir.
2. Bring to the boil, then reduce to a simmer and cook for 25 minutes, or until the bolognese is close to your desired consistency. Add the mushrooms and pumpkin and cook for a further 10–15 minutes, or until the pumpkin is just tender. Remove from the heat and season with salt and pepper.

Mexican Chicken and Easy Guacamole

Spicy and succulent . . . just as chicken should be! If you feel comfortable quartering the chicken yourself, go for it. Otherwise, buy the chicken pieces separately, or even grab a few drumsticks – easier for the kids to enjoy!

SERVES 2-4

1 onion, *sliced*
2 garlic cloves, *chopped*
3 tablespoons olive oil
1 teaspoon smoked paprika
1 teaspoon cumin
½ teaspoon cayenne pepper
½ teaspoon chilli flakes
1 whole chicken, *quartered (or 4-8 chicken pieces)*
sea salt and freshly ground black pepper, to taste
½ bunch of parsley, *chopped*

EASY GUACAMOLE

2 ripe avocados
juice of 1 lime
¼ bunch of coriander, *chopped*
½ teaspoon cumin
sea salt and freshly ground black pepper, to taste

1. Preheat your oven to 180°C.
2. In a large mixing bowl, combine the onion, garlic, oil and spices. Chuck in the chicken and toss to ensure the pieces are well coated.
3. Place the chicken on a baking tray lined with baking paper. Season with salt and pepper then pop in the oven. Bake for 40 minutes, or until cooked through and browned. Remove from the oven and allow to rest for 5 minutes.
4. Meanwhile, combine the ingredients for the guacamole in a mixing bowl. Use a fork and resist mashing the avocado excessively – leave some texture.
5. Serve the guacamole alongside the chicken.

Pan-fried Snapper

This is an awesome go-to recipe for white fish: quick and easy, but a recipe that really celebrates the fish. When in doubt, simply add lemon to a dish (not just with fish!) to bring it to life.

SERVES 2

1 teaspoon butter
½ garlic clove, *minced*
1 long red chilli (optional), *deseeded and chopped*
2 snapper fillets (or John Dory, or hake)
sea salt and freshly ground black pepper, to taste
juice of ½ lemon

1. Place a frying pan over medium heat, add the butter, then add the garlic and chilli, if using, and cook for 1 minute. Season the skin of the fish with salt and pepper. Fry, skin-side down, for 3–4 minutes, or until the skin is crispy. Flip the fish over and cook for a further 2–3 minutes, or until cooked through (cooking times will vary depending on thickness of fillet).
2. Remove from the heat, drizzle with lemon juice, season with more salt and pepper, if desired, and serve.

Meatballs in Tomato Sauce with Baked Pumpkin

This recipe is a favourite with the family and is easy to modify into burgers for the barbecue. When pan-frying the meatballs, the idea is to simply brown and caramelise the meat – the rest of the cooking is done slowly in the tomato sauce.

SERVES 4

500 g pumpkin, *cut into wedges*
1 tablespoon olive oil
½ teaspoon cinnamon
sea salt and freshly ground black pepper, to taste
¼ bunch of parsley leaves, *roughly chopped* (to serve)

MEATBALLS

500 g lamb mince
½ brown onion, *chopped*
2 garlic cloves, *finely chopped*
1 teaspoon Dijon mustard
1 teaspoon paprika
1 teaspoon cumin
¼ bunch of parsley stalks, *chopped*
1 egg yolk
sea salt and freshly ground black pepper, to taste
1 tablespoon butter

TOMATO SAUCE

1 tablespoon olive oil
1 small red onion, *finely chopped*
4 garlic cloves, *finely chopped*
100 ml Beef Bone Broth, optional (see recipe page 246)
1 × 400 g tin chopped tomatoes
100 ml tomato passata
sea salt and freshly ground black pepper, to taste

1. Preheat your oven to 180°C.
2. In a mixing bowl, combine the pumpkin, olive oil and cinnamon, and add salt and pepper to taste. Tip the pumpkin onto a baking tray lined with baking paper, pop in the oven and bake for 35–40 minutes, or until the pumpkin is cooked through and lightly browned.
3. Meanwhile, make the meatballs. In a large mixing bowl, combine the lamb mince with the onion, garlic, mustard, paprika, cumin, parsley stalks and egg yolk. Add salt and pepper to taste. Roll into walnut-sized meatballs and set aside.
4. Now make the tomato sauce. Place a saucepan over medium heat, add the olive oil, then add the onion and garlic and cook for 3–4 minutes, or until softened. Add the beef broth and cook for 1 minute. Add the chopped tomatoes and tomato passata and season with salt and pepper. Cook for a further 20 minutes.
5. Now cook the meatballs. Place a frying pan over medium–high heat, add the butter, then add the meatballs. Cook, turning often, until brown all over.
6. Add the meatballs to the tomato sauce and cook for 5–6 minutes. Remove from the heat, add the parsley leaves, and season with salt and pepper. Serve with the baked pumpkin.

Crispy-skin Sea Trout

SERVES 1

1 sea trout fillet (skin on – optional)
1 teaspoon coconut oil or butter
sea salt and freshly ground black pepper, to taste
juice of ½ lemon

1. Remove the fish from the fridge 30 minutes before cooking.
2. Place a frying pan over high heat and add the oil or butter. Season the skin of the fish with salt and pepper. Fry, skin-side down, for 3–4 minutes, or until the skin is crispy. Flip the fish over and cook for a further 2–3 minutes, or until cooked through (cooking times will vary depending on thickness of fillet). Remove from the heat and allow to rest for 2 minutes. Drizzle with lemon juice, season with extra salt and pepper, if desired, and serve.

Naked Burgers

SERVES 4

4 Portobello mushrooms
2 tablespoons olive oil
½ sprig of rosemary
½ sprig of thyme
2 garlic cloves, *sliced*
sea salt and freshly ground black pepper, to taste
2 garlic cloves, *finely chopped*
500 g beef mince
1 small brown onion, *finely chopped*
1 long red chilli, *deseeded and finely chopped*
1 teaspoon Dijon mustard
1 egg yolk
1 teaspoon cumin
1 teaspoon dried oregano
2 tablespoons butter or coconut oil
Aïoli, to serve (see recipe page 269)

1. Preheat your oven to 180°C.

2. Remove the stems from the mushrooms and drizzle with olive oil. Place on a baking tray lined with baking paper, bottom-side up. Sprinkle with the rosemary, thyme and the sliced garlic. Season with salt and pepper, pop in the oven and bake for 20 minutes, or until softened.

3. Combine the finely chopped garlic, beef mince, onion, chilli, mustard, egg yolk, cumin and oregano. Season with salt and pepper and divide into four patties.

4. Place a frying pan over medium heat and add the butter or coconut oil. Cook the patties for 2–3 minutes on one side, then flip and cook for a further 1–2 minutes or until cooked to your liking. Remove from the heat and allow to rest for 2–3 minutes.

5. To serve, place the patties on a mushroom and top with a spoonful of aïoli.

Poached Salmon with Courgette Ribbons

SERVES 1

1 salmon fillet
2 courgettes, *cut into ribbons or noodles*
handful of cherry tomatoes, *halved*
handful of basil leaves
2 tablespoons olive oil
sea salt and freshly ground black pepper, to taste
squeeze of lemon juice

1. Bring some salted water to the boil in a saucepan. Gently place the fish in the water, pop the lid on and turn the heat off. Leave to stand for 8–10 minutes, depending on the size of the fillet. (Perfectly cooked salmon should flake apart easily and have a beautiful sheen to it. If it's undercooked it won't flake apart, but hold together instead.) Remove from the water and set aside.
2. In a mixing bowl, combine the courgettes, tomato, basil and olive oil. Season with salt and pepper. Break the salmon fillet into the courgette mixture and gently stir through. Add a squeeze of lemon juice and season with more salt and pepper, if desired, and serve.

Poached Chicken in Broth

SERVES 2

1 litre Chicken Bone Broth (see recipe page 247)
300 g chicken thigh meat, *chopped*
2 carrots, *sliced*
2 shallots, *trimmed and chopped*
handful of kale, *trimmed and chopped*
1 teaspoon chilli flakes
1 tablespoon butter
sea salt and freshly ground black pepper, to taste
¼ bunch of parsley, *chopped*

1. Place a saucepan over medium heat and bring the broth up to a simmer. Throw in the chicken, carrots and shallots and cook for 5 minutes. Add the kale and continue to cook for a further 5 minutes, or until the chicken is cooked through. Add the chilli flakes and butter, season with salt and pepper, and remove from the heat. Sprinkle with the parsley to serve.

Grilled Mexican Chicken

SERVES **4**

3 tablespoons butter
2 teaspoons paprika
1 small brown onion, *chopped*
2 garlic cloves, *chopped*
½ teaspoon cayenne pepper
½ teaspoon cumin
1 teaspoon honey
500 g chicken breast, *butterflied*
sea salt and freshly ground black pepper, to taste

1. In a mixing bowl, combine all the ingredients except the chicken and salt and pepper.
2. Heat a griddle or grill. Thoroughly coat the chicken with the spice rub and cook for 4–5 minutes on each side, or until cooked through. Remove from the heat, allow to rest for 5 minutes, then season with salt and pepper and serve.

Baked Salmon in a Bag

SERVES 2

2 baby fennel bulbs, *trimmed, cored and thinly sliced*
200 g cherry tomatoes, *halved*
handful of kalamata olives, *roughly chopped*
2 tablespoons olive oil
2 salmon fillets
1 lemon, *thinly sliced*
½ bunch of dill
sea salt and freshly ground black pepper, to taste

1. Preheat your oven to 160°C.
2. In a mixing bowl, combine the fennel, cherry tomatoes, olives and olive oil. Tip the mix onto a baking tray lined with baking paper and pop in the oven for 30 minutes, or until the vegetables have softened. Remove from the oven and set aside.
3. Cut two large squares of baking paper. Place a salmon fillet in the middle of each piece of paper and top with the sliced lemon. Spoon some of the fennel and tomato mixture over the fish and pop a sprig of dill on top. Season with salt and pepper.
4. Create a parcel by grabbing the four corners of the paper and bringing them together before tying with baking twine. Bake in the oven on a tray for 8–10 minutes, or until the fish is just cooked through. Remove from the oven and allow to rest for 3–4 minutes.
5. Use scissors to cut the tops off the parcels. Serve.

Baked Snapper with Chilli

SERVES **2**

1 tablespoon lemon juice
75 ml lime juice
1 teaspoon chilli flakes
2 snapper fillets (or other firm white fish)
4 spring onions, *chopped*
½ red pepper, *deseeded and diced*
½ yellow pepper, *deseeded and diced*
1 tomato, *diced*
sea salt and freshly ground black pepper, to taste
3–4 tablespoons coriander, *roughly chopped*

1. Preheat your oven to 180°C. Line a baking tray with baking paper.
2. Combine the lemon and lime juice and stir in the chilli. Place the snapper fillets in a glass or ceramic baking dish, pour the marinade over the fillets and leave for 10 minutes.
3. Combine the spring onions, red and yellow peppers and tomato, and sprinkle over the fish. Cover the dish with foil and pop in the oven for 15–20 minutes, or until the fish is cooked through. Remove from the heat and allow to rest for 5 minutes.
4. To serve, season the snapper with salt and pepper, and finish with a sprinkle of chopped coriander.

Hoki in Coconut Broth

SERVES 2

1 tablespoon butter
1 brown onion, *finely chopped*
4 garlic cloves, *finely chopped*
½ bunch of coriander, *stalks finely chopped and leaves roughly chopped*
1 long red chilli (optional), *deseeded and finely chopped*
150 ml chicken or vegetable broth
splash of white wine (optional)
1 tablespoon fish sauce (nam pla)
1 × 400 ml tin coconut cream or milk
500 g hoki (or hake, cod)
juice of ½ lime
sea salt and freshly ground black pepper, to taste

1. Place a large, lidded frying pan over medium heat and add the butter, then add the onion, garlic, coriander stalks and chilli, if using. Cook for 4–5 minutes, or until the onion has softened. Add the broth and white wine, if using, and turn up the heat. Add the fish sauce and coconut cream and stir. Add the hoki and gently stir. Pop the lid on the pan and cook for 5–6 minutes over medium heat.
2. Remove from the heat, squeeze over the lime juice, season with salt and pepper, and serve.

Pan-fried Hake

SERVES **1**

1 tablespoon butter
2 garlic cloves, *sliced*
1 tablespoon capers, *roughly chopped*
2 hake fillets
2 small cucumbers, *diced*
3 tomatoes, *diced*
¼ bunch of basil
juice of ½ lemon
1 tablespoon olive oil
sea salt and freshly ground black pepper, to taste

1. Place a frying pan over medium heat, add the butter, then add the garlic and capers and cook for 1–2 minutes. Add the fish and cook for 2–3 minutes on each side. Remove from the heat.
2. Spoon some of the garlic/caper mixture from the pan onto the fish. Allow to rest for 1 minute.
3. Combine the cucumber, tomato, basil, lemon juice and olive oil. Season with salt and pepper, and serve with the fish.

Whole Baked Snapper with Salsa Verde

A simple yet visually stunning recipe – perfect for a dinner party. You can also use whole sea bass or bream.

SERVES 4

1 whole snapper, *gutted and descaled*
1 bunch of dill
2 lemons, *sliced*
1 bunch of coriander
sea salt and freshly ground black pepper, to taste
2 tablespoons Salsa Verde (see recipe page 151)

1. Preheat your oven to 180°C.
2. Make four or five 1 cm-deep slashes diagonally across the fish, from behind the gills to the tail. Take some dill and insert it into the incisions. Place half the lemon slices into the cavity of the fish, along with the remaining dill and the coriander – you'll need to scrunch the coriander up to get it all in.
3. Place the remaining lemon slices on a baking tray lined with baking paper. Lie the fish on top of the lemon and season with salt and pepper. Pop in the oven and bake for 20–25 minutes, or until the fish is just cooked. Remove from the oven and allow to rest for 5 minutes before serving with a spoonful of salsa verde over the top.

Beef Goulash

My folks used to cook goulash in their pubs when I was a kid.
I still love it to this day.

SERVES 4

1 tablespoon beef dripping or butter
2 brown onions, *roughly chopped*
2 garlic cloves, *roughly chopped*
500 g stewing steak, *diced*
1 large red pepper, *sliced*
1 × 400 g tin diced tomatoes
250 ml tomato passata
500 ml Beef Bone Broth (see recipe page 246)
2 tablespoons paprika
2 teaspoons caraway seeds
sea salt and black pepper, to taste
½ bunch of parsley, *roughly chopped*

1. Place a large, lidded frying pan or saucepan over medium heat and
   add the dripping or butter, then add the onion and garlic and cook
   for 4–5 minutes, or until softened. Turn the heat to high and add
   the steak. Brown off the meat before adding the red pepper, diced
   tomato, tomato passata, beef broth, paprika and caraway seeds.
   Season with salt and pepper.
2. Reduce the heat, pop the lid on and cook over low heat for a further
   45–60 minutes, or until the beef is tender. Remove the lid and
   continue simmering to thicken to your desired consistency. Remove
   from the heat and stir in the parsley.

Butter Chicken

My son Tashi would eat butter chicken every single night, given the choice! This is a simple and quick version of the classic recipe.

SERVES 4

2 tablespoons ghee or butter
6 overripe tomatoes, *roughly chopped*
500 g chicken thigh, *roughly chopped*
1 tablespoon garam masala
1 tablespoon ground coriander
1 tablespoon cumin
1 teaspoon ground chilli
5 cm knob of root ginger, *peeled and finely chopped*
4 garlic cloves, *minced*
1 × 400 ml tin coconut cream
4 tablespoons butter
sea salt and freshly ground black pepper (optional)
¼ bunch of coriander, *chopped*

1. Place a saucepan over medium heat, add the ghee or butter, then add the tomato until it begins to break down and thicken. Add the chicken and the spices and cook for 5 minutes, or until the chicken begins to brown.
2. Reduce the heat and stir in the ginger, garlic and coconut cream. Simmer for 15–20 minutes, or until the sauce has thickened. Remove from the heat and stir the butter through. Season with salt and pepper, and sprinkle with the coriander.

Lamb and Bacon Casserole

Back in the day, I would have baked this with a sweet potato topping. This recipe is still yummy, but more keto-friendly.

SERVES 4

150 g bacon, *chopped*
2 tablespoons butter
1 brown onion, *chopped*
4 garlic cloves, *chopped*
1 leek, *chopped*
500 g lamb mince
1 teaspoon chopped rosemary
1 teaspoon dried oregano
2 × 400 g tins diced tomatoes
150 ml tomato passata
250 ml Beef Bone Broth (see recipe page 246)
sea salt and freshly ground black pepper, to taste

1. Preheat your oven to 180°C.
2. Place a frying pan over medium heat and cook the bacon for 3–4 minutes, or until the fat is rendered. Remove from the pan and set aside.
3. Heat the butter in the pan over medium heat, add the onion, garlic and leek and cook for 3–4 minutes, or until the vegetables begin to soften. Turn the heat up and throw in the lamb mince. Stir until browned. Add the bacon and any residual fat, then add the herbs, diced tomato, tomato passata and broth. Reduce the heat and simmer for 20–25 minutes, or until the casserole has thickened to your liking. Season with salt and pepper.

Steak and Kidney

Folks would flock from miles around for my mum's steak and kidney pie. My version holds true to her recipe, except for the pastry base. If you can't get hold of beef dripping (a rendered form of beef or mutton fat) or lard (rendered or unrendered pig fat), butter or ghee will do just as well.

SERVES 4

2 tablespoons beef dripping or lard
2 onions, *chopped*
4 garlic cloves, *chopped*
400 g stewing steak, *diced*
200 g lamb or beef kidneys, *trimmed and diced*
2 carrots, *chopped*
2 celery sticks, *chopped*
1 teaspoon chopped fresh rosemary
1 teaspoon dried tarragon
1 teaspoon dried or fresh thyme
500 ml Beef Bone Broth (see recipe page 246)
2 × 400 g tins diced tomatoes
150 ml tomato passata
2 bay leaves
handful of brown mushrooms, *quartered*
sea salt and freshly ground black pepper, to taste

1. Place a lidded, heavy-based saucepan over medium heat, add the beef dripping or lard, then add the onion and garlic and sauté for 3–4 minutes. Add the steak and kidney and increase the heat to brown the meat off. Add the carrot, celery, rosemary, tarragon, thyme, beef broth, diced tomatoes and tomato passata. Reduce the heat to a simmer and cook for 90 minutes. Add the bay leaves and mushrooms and pop the lid on. Simmer for a further 90 minutes, or until the beef is tender.
2. Remove the lid and reduce the liquid to a consistency you like. Remove from the heat and season with salt and pepper before serving.

Beef Rendang

This is a beautiful, aromatic dish. Consider making a batch of the paste to save for next time you want to cook this recipe.

SERVES 4

3 tablespoons coconut oil
500 g stewing steak, *diced*
2 × 400 ml tins coconut cream
1 tablespoon tamarind paste
2 tablespoons desiccated coconut (toasted)

PASTE

15 dried chillies (soaked)
6 shallots, *roughly chopped*
2 cm knob of root ginger, *peeled and roughly chopped*
2 cm of galangal, *roughly chopped*
2 stalks of lemongrass, white part only, *roughly chopped*
sea salt and freshly ground pepper, to taste

1. Combine all the paste ingredients in a blender or food processor and blitz until fully combined.
2. Place a heavy-based saucepan over medium heat, add the coconut oil, then add the paste and cook for 4–5 minutes. Toss the beef through with the paste. Cook until brown, then stir in the coconut cream, tamarind paste and toasted coconut. Cook over low heat, stirring occasionally, for 2 hours, or until the beef is tender. Add some water during the cooking process if required.

Mussels in a Coconut Broth

This was a dish I threw together one day with the ingredients I had in the fridge. From memory, the first version used prawns. Any mixed seafood would work well, too.

SERVES 4

1 tablespoon coconut oil
1 red onion, *finely chopped*
4 garlic cloves, *finely chopped*
5 cm knob of root ginger, *finely chopped*
½ bunch of coriander, *stalks finely chopped and leaves roughly chopped*
1 long red chilli (optional), *deseeded and finely chopped*
150 ml chicken or fish broth
1 tablespoon fish sauce (nam pla)
200 g spinach, *roughly chopped*
1 × 400 ml tin coconut cream
500 g mussels
sea salt, to taste
juice of ½ lime

1. Heat a large, lidded frying pan over medium heat, add the coconut oil, then add the onion, garlic, ginger, coriander stalks and chilli and sauté until softened. Add the broth and fish sauce and bring up to a simmer. Stir in the spinach and coconut cream. Add the mussels, coating well with the sauce. Pop the lid on and cook for 5–6 minutes, or until the mussels have opened.
2. Serve in a deep bowl, season to taste, and garnish with the coriander leaves and a squeeze of lime.

Tandoori Chicken

This recipe works just as well on a griddle or a barbecue as it does in the oven.

SERVES 4

4 garlic cloves, *finely chopped*
2 small red chillies, *finely chopped*
5 cm knob of root ginger, *peeled and finely chopped*
1 teaspoon ground coriander
1 teaspoon paprika
1 teaspoon cumin
1 teaspoon turmeric
1 teaspoon garam masala
1 tablespoon ghee
500 g chicken thigh or breast

1. Preheat your oven to 200°C.
2. Combine the garlic, chilli, ginger and spices in a bowl and add the ghee to form a paste. Place the chicken in the bowl and coat well with the marinade. (For best results, cover and place in the fridge for 2 hours.)
3. Line a baking tray with baking paper. Tip the chicken onto the tray and bake for 30 minutes, or until the chicken is browned and cooked through. (If cooking on the barbecue, preheat to medium heat. Cook, turning often, for 25 minutes, or until browned and cooked through.) Allow to rest for 5 minutes before serving.

Irish Beef Stew

More proof that healthy food can be familiar and comforting!

SERVES **4**

1 tablespoon ghee
6 shallots, *peeled and quartered*
6 garlic cloves, *finely chopped*
500 g stewing steak, *diced*
240 ml red wine
240 ml Guinness or other stout
500 ml Beef Bone Broth (see recipe page 246)
1 tablespoon dried parsley
1 tablespoon thyme
2 bay leaves
4 carrots, *sliced*
2–3 celery sticks, *sliced*
sea salt and freshly ground pepper, to taste
¼ bunch of fresh parsley

1. Place a large saucepan over medium heat, add the ghee, then add
   the shallots and garlic and sauté for 2–3 minutes. Turn the heat
   up and add the beef. Cook to brown off, then add the red wine
   and Guinness and allow the alcohol to burn off – about 1 minute.
   Add the broth, herbs, carrot and celery, and season with salt and
   pepper. Turn the heat down to a simmer and pop the lid on. Allow
   to cook for 1½ hours.
2. Remove the lid and allow the sauce to thicken – about 20 minutes.
   Add the fresh parsley before serving.

Moroccan Beef Stew

This is a perfect dish to make in a large quantity and take to work as leftovers during the week. Ras el hanout is a spice blend from North Africa. Commonly used in the blend are cardamom, cumin, nutmeg, mace, coriander, chilli and cloves.

SERVES 4

1 tablespoon ghee
2 onions, *finely chopped*
6 garlic cloves, *finely chopped*
1 teaspoon smoked paprika
1 teaspoon sweet paprika
1 tablespoon ras el hanout
2 teaspoons cumin
500 g stewing steak, *diced*
grated zest of 1 lemon
1 × 400 g tin diced tomatoes
500 ml Beef Bone Broth (see recipe page 246)
400 g red or brown lentils
100 g green olives, *pitted and halved*
sea salt and black pepper, to taste

1. Place a large saucepan over medium heat, add the ghee, then add the onion and garlic and sauté for 2–3 minutes. Add the spices and stir to combine. Increase the heat and add the beef. Once browned off, add the lemon zest, tomato, broth, lentils and olives. Reduce the heat to a simmer, pop the lid on and cook for 1½ hours.
2. Remove the lid and allow the sauce to thicken – about 20 minutes. Season with salt and pepper before serving.

Jerk Chicken

Jerk chicken should be a combination of tang, some sweetness, and heat. This recipe is great done on the barbecue.

SERVES 4

1½ tablespoons allspice
5 cm knob of root ginger, *peeled and roughly chopped*
2 teaspoons cinnamon
3 garlic cloves, *peeled and halved*
2 hot habaneros chillies, *deseeded*
1 tablespoon honey
3 shallots, *roughly chopped*
1 tablespoon dried thyme
juice of 2 limes
2 tablespoons olive oil
500 g chicken thigh or breast
¼ bunch of coriander, *roughly chopped*
sea salt, to taste

1. Combine all the ingredients except the chicken and coriander in a blender and blitz for 20 seconds. Transfer from the blender to a mixing bowl and coat the chicken well. Allow to marinate in the fridge for 2 hours.
2. Preheat the oven to 180°C.
3. Line a baking tray with baking paper. Tip the chicken onto the tray and bake for 40–45 minutes, or until golden and cooked through. Garnish with fresh coriander and season to taste before serving.

Beef Stroganoff

One of my all-time favourite recipes – I thank my folks for this one.

SERVES 4

2 tablespoons ghee
1 onion, *chopped*
2 garlic cloves, *chopped*
500 g stewing steak, *diced*
1 tablespoon dried thyme
1 tablespoon dried rosemary
3 teaspoons Dijon mustard
150 ml white wine
500 ml Beef Bone Broth (see recipe page 246)
150 ml coconut cream
1 tablespoon arrowroot flour
400 g button mushrooms, *halved*
sea salt and freshly ground pepper, to taste

1. Place a large saucepan over medium heat, add the ghee, then add the onion and garlic and sauté for 2–3 minutes.
2. Add the beef and brown off, stirring occasionally until caramelised. Add the herbs to the pan, stir for 1–2 minutes, then add the mustard.
3. Add the wine and allow the alcohol to burn off – about 1 minute. Add the broth, and stir.
4. Add the coconut cream and stir in enough arrowroot flour to thicken to the desired consistency (add more arrowroot if necessary). Cook over low heat for 1 hour, then add the mushrooms. Continue cooking for a further 30 minutes, or until the meat is tender. Remove from the heat, season with salt and pepper, and serve.

Beef Madras

SERVES **4**

1 tablespoon ghee
2 small brown onions, *roughly chopped*
4 garlic cloves, *roughly chopped*
2 red chillies, *deseeded and roughly chopped*
2 tablespoons ground coriander
1 tablespoon cumin
1 teaspoon turmeric
1 teaspoon ground chilli
500 g stewing steak, *diced*
250 ml tomato passata
450 ml Beef Bone Broth (see recipe page 246)
100 ml coconut cream
½ bunch of coriander, *roughly chopped*

1. Place a deep saucepan over medium heat, add the ghee, then add
   the onion, garlic and chilli and cook for 2–3 minutes. Add the spices
   and stir for 1 minute. Add the steak and stir to coat with spices.
   Once the beef is browned, add the tomato passata, beef broth and
   coconut cream. Pop the lid on and reduce the heat to low. Simmer
   for 1 hour, or until the beef is tender, stirring occasionally during
   the cooking process.
2. To thicken the sauce, remove the lid and increase the heat.
   Alternatively, if the curry is too thick, add some water. Remove
   from the heat and garnish with fresh coriander before serving.

Snapper Stew

The foundation of this recipe is a good tomato sauce.

SERVES 4

1 tablespoon ghee
1 red onion, *finely chopped*
2 garlic cloves, *finely chopped*
1 long red chilli, *deseeded and finely chopped*
½ bunch of parsley, *stalks finely chopped*
90 ml fish broth or Chicken Bone Broth (see recipe page 247)
150 ml tomato passata
1 × 400 g tin diced tomatoes
400 g cherry tomatoes
50 g kalamata olives, *pitted and halved*
1 tablespoon capers, *roughly chopped*
6 anchovy fillets, *roughly chopped*
sea salt and freshly ground black pepper, to taste
500 g snapper fillets, or other white fish (e.g. hake, cod)

1. Place a frying pan or saucepan over medium heat, add the ghee, then add the onion, garlic, chilli and parsley stalks. Sauté until softened.
2. Add the broth, tomato passata, diced tomatoes, cherry tomatoes, olives, capers and anchovies, and season with salt and pepper. Cook for 5 minutes to allow the flavours to blend and the sauce to thicken.
3. Reduce the heat to a simmer and throw in the fish fillets. Cook for 3–5 minutes, or until the fish is cooked through.

Beef Cheeks in Chinese Five-spice

I still remember the first time I tried beef cheeks; to this day I reckon they are hard to beat. Cooked well, the fat within the cheeks melts away and the meat falls apart. The flavours of this dish are strong but delicious. Make sure you reduce the broth at the end to make a sticky sauce.

SERVES 4

1 tablespoon lard or butter
4 beef cheeks
1 litre Beef Bone Broth (see recipe page 246)
2 cinnamon sticks
2 star anise
2 teaspoons Chinese five-spice
2 tablespoons honey
4 small brown onions, *peeled and quartered*
2 garlic cloves, *peeled and quartered*
sea salt and freshly ground black pepper, to taste

1. Preheat your oven to 250°C.
2. Place a large frying pan over high heat and add the lard or butter. Throw in the beef cheeks and cook until browned all over. Remove from the heat and place in a casserole dish. Cover with broth and add the spices, honey, onion and garlic. Add more water if necessary (the cheeks should be 90 per cent covered with liquid). Reduce the oven temperature to 140°C and cook with the lid on for 5–6 hours, or until the cheeks fall apart.
3. Drain the liquid off into a saucepan and rapidly reduce over high heat. Once the sauce is reduced, remove from the heat, season with salt and pepper, and serve with the beef cheeks.

Lamb Shank Ragu with Cauli 'n' Broccoli Rice

This recipe works well for shanks or diced lamb leg and can be cooked in a pressure cooker or slow cooker. The lamb will fall apart and combine with the richness of the sauce. Don't be put off by the number of ingredients in this recipe. At the end of the day, it's a one-pot wonder!

SERVES 2-4

1 tablespoon beef dripping or olive oil
4 lamb shanks (or 500 g diced lamb)
200 g pancetta, *roughly chopped*
1 litre Beef Bone Broth (see recipe page 246)
200 ml tomato passata
2 × 400 g tins diced tomatoes
4 small brown onions, *peeled and quartered*
4 garlic cloves, *roughly chopped*
40 g anchovies, *finely chopped*
1 bunch of parsley, *stalks finely chopped*
1 bunch of oregano, *roughly chopped*
1 tablespoon butter
¼ head of cauliflower, *roughly chopped*
¼ head of broccoli, *roughly chopped*
sea salt and freshly ground black pepper, to taste

1. Preheat your oven to 250°C.
2. Place a large frying pan over high heat and add the beef dripping or coconut oil, then add the lamb. Fry until until browned off. Transfer to a casserole and pour in any pan juices. Deglaze the pan with some water and add this to the pot too.
3. Fry the pancetta until the fat is rendered. Throw in with the lamb. Cover the lamb with the beef broth, tomato passata, diced tomatoes, onion, garlic, anchovies, parsley stalks and oregano. Season lightly with salt and pepper. Pop the lid on, reduce the oven temperature to 140°C and bake for 3 hours, or until lamb falls away from the bone.
4. Throw the cauliflower and broccoli in a large blender, or do in batches if your blender is small. Process on a low setting until the veggies resemble rice.
5. Melt the butter in a large frying pan over high heat, then add the cauliflower and broccoli 'rice'. Toss until the vegetables begin to soften (about 3–4 minutes), then remove from the heat and season with salt and pepper. (It's also possible to serve the cauliflower and broccoli rice raw – simply dress with some olive/nut oil and season with salt and pepper.) Serve the veggie rice with the lamb shanks.

Pork Belly with Braised Cabbage

Pork belly is my favourite menu choice when eating out in a restaurant. There are few things better in life than crispy pork crackling.

1 teaspoon cumin seeds
1 teaspoon fennel seeds
4 garlic cloves, *finely chopped*
2 tablespoons coconut oil
½ teaspoon nutmeg
1 kg pork belly
sea salt and freshly ground black pepper, to taste
750 ml Beef Bone Broth (see recipe page 246) or vegetable broth
1 tablespoon mixed peppercorns
¼ white cabbage, *finely shredded*
¼ red cabbage, *finely shredded*
1 tablespoon butter
drizzle of olive oil

1. Preheat your oven to 220°C.
2. In a mortar and pestle, crush the cumin and fennel seeds, then add the garlic, coconut oil and nutmeg. Combine thoroughly.
3. Score the pork belly fat diagonally at 2 cm intervals. Now score the pork a little deeper, cutting right through the fat. This will make serving the crackling after cooking much easier. Rub the spice mix onto the skin and into the score lines to ensure the flavour penetrates the meat. Season with salt and pepper. Place the pork on a baking tray and pop in the oven for 10 minutes. Reduce the heat to 160°C and cook for a further 1½ hours. When cooked, remove and allow to rest for 10 minutes.
4. Pour the broth in a saucepan and add the peppercorns. Bring to the boil, then add the cabbage. Add some water if you need to, to cover the cabbage. Reduce the heat and allow to simmer for 5 minutes, or until the cabbage has softened. Drain and remove from the heat. Add the butter and olive oil, and season with salt and pepper.
5. Slice the pork belly, break up the crackling and serve with the cabbage.

Chilli Con Carne with Avo and Toms

Traditional chilli con carne calls for kidney beans. This is a keto-friendly version, but feel free to add a handful of beans if you wish. Beans are a valuable source of prebiotics, but they do have a higher carb content.

SERVES 4

1 tablespoon ghee
1 brown onion, *finely diced*
2 garlic cloves, *minced*
1 long red chilli, *deseeded (optional) and finely chopped*
1 teaspoon cumin
1 teaspoon dried oregano
2 teaspoons sweet paprika
1 teaspoon cacao powder
500 g beef mince
500 ml Beef Bone Broth (see recipe page 246)
150 ml tomato passata
1 × 400 g tin diced tomatoes
sea salt and freshly ground black pepper, to taste
2 fresh tomatoes, *chopped*
1 avocado, *chopped*
½ bunch of coriander, *chopped*
juice of 1 lime

1. Place a large frying pan or saucepan over medium heat, add the ghee, then add the onion, garlic and chilli. Sauté for 2 minutes. Add the cumin, oregano, paprika and cacao and cook for another 2 minutes, then add the mince and turn up the heat to high to brown it off.

2. Reduce the heat to a simmer and add the beef broth, tomato passata and tinned tomatoes. Season with salt and pepper and leave to simmer until it begins to thicken – about 30–40 minutes. Remove from the heat and set aside.

3. In a bowl, combine the fresh tomatoes, avocado, coriander and lime juice. Season with salt and pepper, and serve with the chilli con carne.

Vegetarian Moroccan Casserole

A warming casserole packed full of flavour and health benefits. If you wanted to add more chickpeas for your post-workout meals, feel free.

SERVES 4

2 tablespoons olive oil
1 large onion, *roughly chopped*
3 garlic cloves, *chopped*
2 cm knob of root ginger, *peeled and minced*
1 tablespoon cinnamon
1 teaspoon cumin
1 tablespoon turmeric
3 teaspoons dried harissa
1 × 400 g tin diced tomatoes
juice of 1 lemon
3–4 tablespoons chopped coriander leaves
3–4 tablespoons chopped mint leaves
300 g pumpkin, *chopped*
3–4 carrots, *chopped*
3–4 courgettes, *chopped*
200 g tinned chickpeas, *rinsed and drained*

1. Preheat your oven to 150°C.
2. Place a casserole dish over medium heat and add the oil, then add the onion and garlic and sauté for 3–4 minutes. Add the ginger and spices and stir to combine. Add the harissa, tomatoes, lemon juice and herbs and bring to the boil. Reduce the heat to a simmer, add the pumpkin, carrot and courgettes, stir well and pop the lid on. Cook for 1 hour in the oven.
3. Add the chickpeas and continue to cook for 5 minutes. Serve.

Vegetarian Korma

This curry lends itself very nicely to white fish. Feel free to add some hake or hake fillets.

SERVES 4

2 tablespoons coconut oil
1 onion, *finely chopped*
3 cardamon pods, *bashed*
2 teaspoons cumin
2 teaspoons ground coriander
½ teaspoon turmeric
1 green chilli, *deseeded and finely chopped*
2 cm knob of root ginger, *peeled and minced*
1 garlic clove, *finely chopped*
2–3 courgettes, *sliced*
300 g pumpkin, *chopped*
½ head of cauliflower, *cut into small florets*
500 ml vegetable broth
200 ml coconut cream
50 g toasted flaked almond

1. Place a large saucepan over low heat and add the oil, then add the onion and spices and cook for 3–4 minutes. Add the chilli, ginger and garlic and cook for 2–3 minutes. Add the courgettes, pumpkin and cauliflower and stir to ensure the veggies are coated in spices. Cook for a further 5 minutes. Add the broth and coconut cream. Continue to cook until the sauce reduces to your desired consistency.
2. Remove from the heat, garnish with toasted almond flakes and serve.

Quick and Easy Lamb

This recipe is incredibly easy and is ready to throw in the oven in no time. Depending how rare you like your lamb, it can be removed from the oven after just 20 minutes. I've used this recipe for dinner parties but also as a 'snack' – and no, I don't eat the whole thing, I just cut off slices and refrigerate the rest for the next day.

SERVES **4**

2 tablespoons olive oil
1.2 kg rolled lamb loin (not trimmed of fat)
2 brown onions, *peeled and quartered*
2 garlic bulbs, *halved*
sea salt and freshly ground black pepper, to taste
juice of ½ lemon

1. Preheat your oven to 220 °C.
2. Place a frying pan over medium–high heat and add the olive oil. Place the lamb in the pan and seal the meat on all sides. Transfer to a casserole dish and scrape in any fat from the pan. Add the onion and place the garlic bulbs, cut-side down, in the oil (add some more oil if you need to). Season the lamb with salt and pepper and pop the lid on the dish. Reduce the oven temperature to 180°C and cook the lamb for 20–25 minutes (rare) or 25–30 minutes (medium).
3. Remove the lamb from the oven cover with foil and allow to rest for 5–10 minutes. Squeeze the lemon over and season with salt and pepper before serving.

Whole Baked Fish

This is a great, versatile recipe to have up your sleeve. It will work with an array of whole fish (trout, mackerel, bass or bream) and will cook nicely on a barbecue as well as in the oven.

SERVES 2 (OR MORE, DEPENDING HOW BIG THE FISH IS)

2 tablespoons butter, plus 1 tablespoon extra
1 bream or sea bass, *gutted and descaled*
2 garlic cloves, *lightly crushed*
2 bay leaves
sprig of thyme
handful of parsley
150 ml dry white wine
juice of 1 lemon
sea salt and freshly ground black pepper, to taste

1. Preheat your oven to 190°C.
2. Rip off a piece of foil large enough to create a parcel to encase the whole fish. Rub 1 tablespoon of butter on the inside of the foil. Place the fish in the middle and insert the garlic, bay leaves, thyme and parsley into the cavity. Pour the wine in, squeeze the lemon juice over, and season with salt and pepper.
3. Close the parcel by scrunching the foil together over the fish. Pop in the oven and bake for 20–25 minutes, or until the fish is just cooked through. Remove from the oven and open up the parcel. Allow to rest for 5 minutes before serving.

Chicken One-pot

A one-pot meal is the height of simplicity. This is a recipe that you'll have on the hob in 10 minutes or less, freeing up the evening for whatever else you wish to do.

SERVES 4

1 chicken
2 brown onions, *peeled and halved*
4 garlic cloves, *peeled and lightly smashed*
1 leek, *trimmed and chopped*
4 carrots, *ends trimmed and chopped*
2 bay leaves
2 celery sticks
bunch of thyme
1 teaspoon peppercorns
¼ bunch of parsley
1 teaspoon sea salt

1. Place the chicken in a large stockpot and cover with water. Bring to the boil, then reduce the heat to a simmer for 35 minutes. Skim off any scum that rises to the top of the broth.
2. Add the remaining ingredients and return to a simmer for a further 30 minutes. Check to see that the chicken is completely cooked.
3. To serve, remove the veggies from the pot and place into a bowl. Remove the whole chicken, place on top of the veggies and pour over some of the broth.

Barbecue Prawns

Nothing screams summer quite like barbecued prawns. This is so easy, and can also work with lobster. The butter can be used to baste the prawns as well as to apply to the cooked prawns. I prefer to cook prawns with their heads on, to add more flavour, but you can use trimmed, butterflied prawns if you prefer.

SERVES 4

120 g salted butter
3 garlic cloves, *finely chopped*
1 long red chilli, *deseeded and roughly chopped*
½ bunch of fresh parsley, *chopped*
24 large raw prawns
juice of 1 lemon
sea salt and freshly ground black pepper, to taste

1. Preheat the barbecue to medium.
2. Place a frying pan over low–medium heat on the hob and add the butter. Heat for 2 minutes, then add the garlic and chilli and cook for a further 2 minutes. Add the parsley and cook for a further minute. Remove the pan from the heat but keep warm.
3. Throw the prawns on the barbecue. Using a brush, smear some of the butter from the pan onto the prawns as they cook, ensuring both sides are covered. Cook for 1–2 minutes each side, or until cooked through, then remove from the barbecue and coat with more of the herb butter and a drizzle of lemon juice. Season with salt and pepper.

Fuss-free Lamb Mince

This is a simple recipe than can easily transfer to beef or chicken mince. Mince is an affordable cut and is super-versatile. It's also a good way of accommodating some veggies into your meals for kids, and is great for making a large batch and eating throughout the week.

SERVES 4

1 tablespoon butter or ghee
1 large brown onion, *chopped*
4 garlic cloves, *chopped*
1 teaspoon cumin seeds
1 teaspoon fennel seeds
500 g lamb mince
500 ml Beef Bone Broth (see recipe page 246)
200 g tender-stem broccoli, *trimmed and chopped (include some stalk)*
bunch of asparagus, *trimmed and chopped into pieces (include some stalk)*
sea salt and freshly ground black pepper, to taste
juice of ½ lemon

1. Place a deep frying pan or saucepan over medium heat, add the butter or ghee, then add the onion, garlic, cumin seeds and fennel seeds and cook for 3–4 minutes, or until the onion starts to soften.
2. Turn the heat up to high, add the mince and brown off, stirring often. Reduce the heat to low and add the broth. Cook for 15 minutes before adding the broccoli and asparagus. Cook for a further 5–10 minutes, or until the veggies are cooked but still a little crunchy. Season with salt and pepper, stir in the lemon juice, and serve.

Liver and Onions

SERVES **4**

2 tablespoons ghee
2 brown onions, *sliced*
2 garlic cloves, *roughly chopped*
400–500 g beef livers, whole or diced
sea salt and freshly ground black pepper, to taste

1. Place a frying pan over medium heat, add half the ghee, then add the onion and garlic and sauté for 4–5 minutes. Remove from the heat and set aside.
2. Return the pan to a high heat, add the remaining ghee, then add the liver and cook for 3 minutes on each side, or until cooked to your liking. For the last minute, throw the onions back in with the liver. Remove from the heat, season with salt and pepper, and serve.

SIDES, SNACKS AND DRINKS

Roasted Bone Marrow with Chimichurri

Bone marrow is one of the most nutrient-dense foods on the planet, rich in omega 3 and DHA, but it's not been included here purely for its nutritional benefits. If you're looking for a delicious entrée or even a decadent snack, then this recipe is the bomb. Ask your butcher to cut up the marrow bones for you.

SERVES 4

8–12 beef bones with marrow, *cut into sections or cut lengthways*
2 tablespoons olive oil
sea salt and freshly ground black pepper, to taste

CHIMICHURRI

½ bunch of coriander
½ bunch of parsley
3–5 mint leaves
1 long green chilli
5 tablespoons olive oil
2 tablespoons red wine vinegar
sea salt and freshly ground black pepper, to taste

1. Preheat your oven to 220°C.
2. Place the marrow bones on a baking tray, drizzle with olive oil, and season with salt and pepper. Pop in the oven for 15 minutes, or until the bones begin to bubble.
3. Meanwhile, throw all the ingredients for the chimichurri in a blender and blitz for 20 seconds, or until fully combined.
4. Remove the bones from the oven and allow to cool for a couple of minutes. Serve with the chimichurri.

Baked Brussels Sprouts with Tahini

SERVES 2

200 g Brussels sprouts, *trimmed and halved*
2 tablespoons ghee
1 teaspoon paprika
1 teaspoon chilli flakes
sea salt and freshly ground black pepper, to taste
squeeze of lemon
2 tablespoons tahini

1. Preheat your oven to 190°C.
2. Place the Brussels sprouts in a mixing bowl and add the ghee and spices. Season with salt and pepper and stir to coat. Tip the Brussels sprouts onto a baking tray lined with baking paper. Pop in the oven and bake for 25–30 minutes, or until the outer leaves are crispy.
3. To serve, squeeze lemon juice over the Brussels sprouts and drizzle with tahini.

Sautéed Kale

Kale is a powerhouse of health – packed full of magnesium and vitamins A, C and K. It's a great addition to a smoothie, to omelettes and to stews.

SERVES **2**

2 tablespoons coconut oil or ghee
200 g kale, *trimmed and roughly chopped*
splash of olive oil or avocado oil
juice of ½ lemon
sea salt and freshly ground black pepper, to taste

1. Place a large frying pan over medium heat, add the coconut oil or ghee, then throw in the kale and lightly toss to ensure the fat coats the leaves. Sauté for 4–5 minutes, or until softened. Remove from the heat, drizzle with the olive oil and lemon juice, and season with salt and pepper.

Veggie Medley

This is an Italian-inspired veggie side. Make a large batch to last the week for school lunches or work.

SERVES 2

1 tablespoon butter or ghee
1 brown onion, *roughly chopped*
2 garlic cloves, *roughly chopped*
3 large tomatoes, *roughly chopped*
2 courgettes, *cut into 1 cm slices*
1 red pepper, *deseeded and roughly chopped*
1 yellow pepper, *deseeded and roughly chopped*
1 teaspoon dried or fresh oregano
1 teaspoon dried or fresh thyme
4 tablespoons olive oil
sea salt and freshly ground black pepper, to taste

1. Place a lidded frying pan over low heat, add the butter or ghee, then add the onion and garlic and sauté for 2–3 minutes, or until they begin to soften. Add the tomato, courgettes, peppers, oregano, thyme and olive oil.
2. Pop the lid on the pan and cook for 8–10 minutes, stirring occasionally. Once the veggies have softened, remove from the heat and season with salt and pepper.

Broccoli/Cauliflower Rice

A low-carb alternative to rice or quinoa.

SERVES 2

½ head of broccoli, *trimmed and cut into small florets*
½ head of cauliflower, *trimmed and cut into small florets*
1 tablespoon butter
macadamia or olive oil, to drizzle
sea salt and freshly ground black pepper, to taste

1. Place the broccoli in a food processor or blender. If using a blender, ensure the speed is on slow and that you don't overpack the jug, otherwise the broccoli will turn to mush. When the broccoli resembles rice, remove from the food processor/blender.
2. Repeat this process with the cauliflower. Combine the broccoli and cauliflower in a mixing bowl and gently toss.
3. Place a large frying pan over medium heat, add the butter, then add the broccoli and cauliflower and cook for 6 minutes, gently tossing. Remove from the heat, drizzle with oil and season with salt and pepper.

Baked Whole Cauliflower

This recipe is super-easy and quite a showstopper at dinner parties.

SERVES 6

60 g butter, ghee or olive oil
2 garlic cloves, *roughly chopped*
1 teaspoon grated lemon zest
1 teaspoon cumin
1 head of cauliflower, *stalk and leaves trimmed*
sea salt and freshly ground black pepper, to taste

1. Preheat your oven to 180°C.
2. In a mixing bowl, combine the fat with the garlic, lemon zest and cumin.
3. Place the cauliflower in a baking dish lined with baking paper. Pour the oil mixture over the top and season with salt and pepper. Cover with a lid or foil and pop in the oven for 1¼ hours, or until the cauliflower is cooked through. Remove from the heat and baste the cauliflower with the juices in the tray.

Raw Kale Slaw

This is a great addition to many a meal. Feel free to add a tahini dressing or vinaigrette.

SERVES 2

100 g kale, *finely chopped*
1 carrot, *cut into matchsticks*
1 fennel, *trimmed, cored and cut into matchsticks*
sea salt and freshly ground black pepper, to taste

1. In a bowl, combine the kale, carrot and fennel. Add a dressing, if using one. Season with salt and pepper.

Nearly Colcannon

I feel I was late to the party with this dish, having only come across it a few years ago at Colin Fassnidge's restaurant in Sydney. A classic Irish veggie dish, it's affordable and, doused in butter, tastes unreal. Genuine colcannon is potato mash with cabbage, but my recipe is just buttery cabbage. It makes for a great side dish.

100 g salted butter
½ Savoy cabbage, shredded
sea salt and freshly ground black pepper, to taste
juice of ¼ lemon

1. Place a large frying pan over low heat, and add the butter and stir until melted. Add the cabbage and stir to ensure it is coated in the butter. Cook for 6–8 minutes, or until the cabbage has softened. Season with salt and pepper, and add a squeeze of lemon before serving.

Mushrooms in Butter and Thyme

This is a recipe I've been making for 30 years. As a kid I remember throwing some mushrooms in a bowl with butter and chucking it in the microwave. Next minute: buttery mushrooms on toast! Here's the latest version.

SERVES 2

2 tablespoons butter or ghee
½ sprig of thyme
2–3 large handfuls of chopped mushrooms
sea salt and freshly ground black pepper, to taste

1. Place a large frying pan over low–medium heat, add the butter to melt, then add the thyme and heat for 1 minute. Add the mushrooms and cook for 7–10 minutes, stirring occasionally.
2. Once the mushrooms have softened, remove the pan from the heat, season with salt and pepper, and serve.

Heirloom Tomato Salad

I absolutely love the shapes and colours of heirloom tomatoes. They also offer an almost meat-like component to the dish, being so succulent.

SERVES 2

4 heirloom tomatoes, *sliced*
1 avocado, *sliced*
4 anchovy fillets
olive oil or avocado oil
handful of basil leaves, *roughly torn*
sea salt and freshly ground black pepper, to taste

1. Combine the tomato, avocado and anchovy fillets (roughly chopped if you prefer) in a bowl. Dress with oil, toss in the basil leaves and season with salt and pepper.

All the Greens

3 tablespoons butter
2 garlic cloves, *chopped*
3 shallots, *chopped*
1 large leek, *chopped*
handful of Brussels sprouts, *trimmed and roughly chopped*
100 ml Chicken Bone Broth (see recipe page 247)
¼ bunch of parsley, *chopped*
sea salt and freshly ground black pepper, to taste
2 tablespoons Salsa Verde (see recipe page 151)

1. Place a frying pan over medium heat, add the butter, then add the garlic and shallots and cook for 2–3 minutes. Add the leek and Brussels sprouts and cook for 6–8 minutes, or until the Brussels sprouts begin to soften. Add the broth and cook for another 1–2 minutes. Toss through the parsley, remove from the heat and season with salt and pepper. Top with salsa verde and serve.

Roasted Veggies with Tahini Dressing

Just because you're aiming for low carb doesn't mean starchy carbs are completely out the window. A recipe with some higher-carb veggies might work well on your training days if you're engaging in cyclic keto.

SERVES 4

2 swedes, *roughly chopped*
4 garlic heads, *halved crossways*
4 carrots, *roughly chopped*
½ head of cauliflower, *cut into small florets*
2 fennel bulbs, *trimmed, cored and thinly sliced*
4 red onions, *peeled and halved*
3 sprigs of rosemary
3 sprigs of thyme
3 tablespoons beef dripping or lard
sea salt, to taste

TAHINI DRESSING

1 tablespoon tahini
½ garlic clove, *finely chopped*
juice of 1 lemon
splash of water
½ teaspoon cumin
sea salt and freshly ground black pepper, to taste

1. Preheat the oven to 180°C.
2. In a large mixing bowl, combine the veggies and herbs with the beef dripping or lard. Gently toss to ensure the veggies are well coated in the fat and herbs. Season with salt.
3. Line a baking tray with baking paper and tip the veggies onto it. Pop in the oven and roast for 35–40 minutes, or until the veggies are softened and golden. Season with salt and pepper.
4. Combine all the ingredients for the tahini dressing. Adjust the amount of water to reach the consistency you like. Serve the veggies with the dressing drizzled on top.

Chicken Liver Pâté

Growing up in pubs in the UK, I was exposed to foods that my peers didn't necessarily know about, like oxtail, liver, kidney and pâté. Pâté was a regular in my lunchbox – today the smell and taste of it always evokes fond memories. I hope you enjoy this recipe as much as I do.

MAKES ABOUT 450 G

115 g butter (or the equivalent in beef dripping, bacon fat or coconut oil)
1 small brown onion, *finely chopped*
2–3 garlic cloves, *minced*
400 g chicken livers, *trimmed of sinew or discoloured bits*
1 sprig of rosemary
2 sprigs of thyme
¼ teaspoon nutmeg
1 teaspoon Dijon mustard
1 teaspoon lemon juice
75 ml Beef Bone Broth (see recipe page 246)
150 ml red wine
sea salt and freshly ground black pepper, to taste

1. Place a frying pan over medium heat, add a tablespoon of the butter and sauté the onion, garlic and liver until the livers are browned and the onions are softened. Add the rosemary, thyme, nutmeg, mustard, lemon juice, broth and wine and cook over low heat until the liquid has evaporated. Remove from the heat.
2. Transfer to a food processor and blend whilst adding the butter (melted if preferred) until a smooth consistency is reached. Season to taste with salt and pepper. Transfer to a shallow dish or ramekins and pop in the fridge for 2–3 hours. You can top with a little warmed butter or coconut oil, if you like; both will form an airtight seal once chilled.

Beef Bone Broth

Broth is the backbone of many of my 'wet' dishes. Ask your local butcher for some bones – the more connective tissue, the better.

MAKES 4 LITRES

2–3 kg beef bones
4½ litres water
90 ml apple cider vinegar
4 carrots, *roughly chopped*
2 celery sticks, *roughly chopped*
2 brown onions, *peeled and quartered*
4 garlic cloves, *peeled*
1 tablespoon peppercorns
1 bunch of thyme
2 bay leaves
sea salt and freshly ground black pepper, to taste

1. Preheat your oven to 220°C.
2. Put the bones into a baking tray, season with salt and pepper, and pop in the oven for 30 minutes. When cooked, place the bones and any juices into a large saucepan or stockpot. Add the remaining ingredients, cover the contents with water and bring to the boil. Turn the heat down and simmer for 12 hours.
3. Allow the broth to cool slightly before staining and pouring the liquid into airtight containers. Store the cooled broth in the fridge for 7–10 days or the freezer for 6–12 months.

Chicken Bone Broth

Broths form the base of so many classic recipes, so having a good chicken bone broth recipe up your sleeve is essential.

MAKES **4** LITRES

2 kg chicken carcass or mix of bones and feet
4½ litres water
1 brown onion, *quartered*
4 celery sticks, *roughly chopped*
2 large carrots, *roughly chopped*
1 garlic head, *halved*
2 tablespoons apple cider vinegar
½ bunch of fresh parsley
2 bay leaves
sea salt and freshly ground black pepper, to taste

1. Place all the ingredients in a large stockpot. Bring to the boil, then reduce to a simmer and cook for 12 hours. Turn off the heat and allow to cool. Season to taste.
2. Sieve the ingredients and store the cooled broth in an airtight container in the fridge for 7–10 days or the freezer for 6–12 months.

Vegetable Broth

Having a veggie broth recipe is important – using different broths can change the flavour profile of any dish.

MAKES 4 LITRES

4½ litres water
1 brown onion, *quartered*
4 celery sticks, *roughly chopped*
2 large carrots, *roughly chopped*
1 garlic head, *halved*
2 tablespoons apple cider vinegar
½ bunch of fresh parsley
2 bay leaves
sea salt and freshly ground black pepper, to taste

1. Place all the ingredients in a large stockpot. Bring to the boil then reduce to a simmer and cook for 12 hours. Turn off the heat and allow to cool. Season to taste.
2. Strain the ingredients and store the cooled broth in an airtight container in the fridge for 7–10 days or freezer for 6–12 months.

Roasted Rosemary Macadamias

These suckers are incredibly moreish . . . be warned!

MAKES **250** G

2 large handfuls of raw macadamias
1–2 tablespoons coconut oil
2 tablespoons finely chopped fresh rosemary
1 teaspoon sea salt

1. Combine all the ingredients in a mixing bowl.
2. Heat a frying pan over high heat. Add the nut mixture and cook for 3–4 minutes, tossing often to ensure even 'roasting'. Remove from the heat. When cool, store in an airtight container.

Dips

Homemade dips are a quick and simple way to snack on nutrient-rich foods. Simply store any leftovers in the fridge and you've got the means of making the humble veg a little sexier.

PESTO

1 bunch of basil, *leaves picked*
¼ bunch of mint, *leaves picked*
½ garlic clove roughly chopped
60 g macadamias
75 ml olive oil or avocado oil (or more if needed)
sea salt and freshly ground black pepper, to taste

1. Throw all the ingredients in a blender or food processor. Blitz for 20–30 seconds, or until fully combined. Add more oil if required.

TAPENADE

120 g kalamata olives, *pitted*
1 garlic clove roughly chopped
4 anchovy fillets
1 tablespoon baby capers
75 ml cup olive oil

1. Throw all the ingredients in a blender or food processor. Blitz for 20–30 seconds, or until fully combined.

BABA GANOUSH

2 large aubergines
2 garlic cloves, roughly chopped
juice of ½ lemon (or more if needed)
2 tablespoons tahini
3 teaspoons olive oil (or more if needed)
1 teaspoon cumin
sea salt and freshly ground black pepper, to taste

1. Preheat your oven to 200°C.
2. Pierce several holes in the skin of the aubergines. Place on a baking tray and pop in the oven for 40 minutes, or until the inside has softened. Remove from the oven and allow to cool.
3. Cut the aubergines in half lengthways, scoop out the flesh and place in a food processor. Add the remaining ingredients and blitz for 20–30 seconds, or until fully combined. Add more lemon juice or oil according to taste.

Fat Green Smoothie

A delicious recipe combining one of nature's superfoods, kale, along with some healthy fats. Feel free to substitute nut butter for tahini. If you go down the nut butter route, try making your own with the most healthful of nuts: walnuts, macadamias and pecans.

SERVES 1-2

270 ml coconut cream
1 tablespoon tahini
1 tablespoon coconut butter
½ avocado
1 tablespoon MCT oil
2 tablespoons chocolate or vanilla protein powder
handful of kale or spinach
handful of ice

1. Throw all the ingredients in a blender and blitz for 20–30 seconds, or until fully combined. Pour into a glass (or glasses) and serve.

High-octane Coffee

A very straightforward recipe but one you'll be grateful for . . . the MCT and coffee light up the brain, and the butter combines with the caffeine molecules to give you a rich 'latte-like' result.

SERVES 1

250 ml black coffee
1 tablespoon butter
1 tablespoon MCT oil

1. Place all the ingredients in a blender and blitz for 10 seconds. Pour into a cup and serve.

Choc Delight

The days of milk, banana and honey smoothies are slowly being overshadowed by more nutrient-dense, higher-fat, healthier versions – and this recipe is no different. It is naturally sweetened by the coconut cream.

SERVES 1–2

270 ml coconut cream
small handful of macadamias
½ ripe avocado, *flesh scooped out*
2 tablespoons cacao powder
1 tablespoon tahini or nut butter
½ teaspoon vanilla extract
2 tablespoons MCT oil
handful of ice

1. Place all the ingredients in a blender and blitz for 20 seconds, or until combined. Pour into a glass (or glasses) and serve.

Powerhouse Smoothie

SERVES 2

bunch of kale, *leaves only*
4 rainbow chard or Swiss chard leaves
200 g spinach
1 large tomato
2 carrots
1 apple
1 avocado, *flesh scooped out*
750 ml coconut or almond milk
100 g berries of your choice (fresh or frozen)
handful of ice

1. Throw all the ingredients in a blender and blitz for 20 seconds, or until smooth. Pour into glasses and serve.

The Fat Bomb

This is a staple in my household – a fat-rich smoothie with some greens.

SERVES 1

200 ml coconut cream
1 tablespoon tahini
1 teaspoon MCT oil
2 tablespoons protein powder
handful of kale
2 tablespoons chia seeds
50 ml bone broth (optional)
handful of ice

1. Throw all the ingredients in a blender and blitz for 20 seconds, or until fully combined. Pour into a glass and serve.

Spiced Latte

This little number is a warming delight, as well as being good for you. Turmeric is a powerful anti-inflammatory but also stimulates the growth of new neurones through the BDNF hormone, which elicits new neurons in the memory centre of the brain.

SERVES 2

400 ml coconut cream
100 ml water
1 cinnamon stick
1 star anise
½ teaspoon turmeric
½ teaspoon allspice (optional)
½ teaspoon honey

1. Place a saucepan over low heat and add all the ingredients. Bring to a simmer and continue to heat for 5 minutes to allow the spices to infuse. Add more water if you need to. Pour into mugs (leaving the whole spices in the pan).

Green Goddess

This wouldn't be a legitimate health book if it didn't include a green smoothie – so here it is!

SERVES 1

200 ml coconut milk
½ avocado, *flesh scooped out and frozen*
1 teaspoon maca powder
1 teaspoon honey
70 g kale
1 teaspoon spirulina
handful of ice

1. Throw all the ingredients in a blender and blitz for 20 seconds, or until smooth. Pour into a glass and serve.

Kick Start

Combining your morning coffee with your smoothie kills two birds with one stone. We are all pushed for time in the morning, so this recipe is great for efficiency.

SERVES 1-2

1 espresso shot
1 tablespoon coconut oil
40 g chocolate protein powder
200 ml coconut milk
50 g raw macadamias
½ banana, *frozen*

1. Throw all the ingredients in a blender and blitz for 20 seconds, or until smooth. Pour into a glass and serve.

Gut-healing Smoothie

Don't be alarmed at seeing broth in my smoothie recipes (and don't worry, it won't reek of beef) – it's just a little hack to get some important amino acids into your system.

SERVES 1–2

200 ml coconut cream
50 ml frozen Beef Bone Broth (see recipe page 246)
½ avocado, *flesh scooped out and frozen*
50 ml coconut kefir
40 g vanilla protein powder
1 tablespoon coconut oil
50 g raw macadamias
handful of ice

1. Throw all the ingredients in a blender and blitz for 20 seconds, or until smooth. Pour into a glass and serve.

Matcha Minty

Naturally occurring in veggies and some fruits, chlorophyll is a potent antioxidant and can bind to toxic heavy metals to help detoxification. It is available in most health food shops or online. The mint leaves certainly lift this thick, refreshing smoothie.

SERVES 1–2

200 ml coconut cream
50 ml matcha green tea
1 teaspoon chlorophyll
½ avocado, *flesh scooped out and frozen*
½ small cucumber
⅓ banana, *frozen*
4–6 fresh mint leaves
1 teaspoon cacao nibs
handful of ice

1. Throw all the ingredients in a blender and blitz for 20 seconds, or until smooth. Pour into a glass and serve.

Post-workout Smoothie

Creatine is an organic phosphate required in the production of energy. Available in health food shops and online, supplementing with creatine can aid recovery and improve subsequent output. Glutamine is the most abundant amino acid in the body – a building block for protein, it aids gut function, immunity and general repair. It's also available in most health food shops and online.

SERVES **1–2**

200 ml coconut cream
1–2 tablespoons vanilla or chocolate protein powder
⅓ banana, *frozen*
1 teaspoon creatine
1 teaspoon glutamine
1 teaspoon cinnamon
1 tablespoon nut butter of your choice
handful of ice

1. Throw all the ingredients in a blender and blitz for 20 seconds, or until smooth. Pour into a glass and serve.

Prebiotic Smoothie

One of the world's richest sources of gut-feeding, resistant starch is the Jerusalem artichoke. They're those funny-looking knobbly things that look a bit like root ginger but are most reminiscent of the potato. Start throwing some of these into your shopping basket from here on in – they're affordable and they pack a punch from a health perspective.

SERVES 1-2

200 ml coconut cream
1 tablespoon nut butter of your choice
2 tablespoons chocolate or vanilla protein powder
½ Jerusalem artichoke, *roughly chopped*
1 tablespoon hemp seeds
small handful of baby spinach
handful of ice

1. Throw all the ingredients in a blender and blitz for 20 seconds, or until smooth. Pour into a glass and serve.

Bulletproof Matcha Green Tea

Matcha is an incredibly powerful antioxidant and anti-ageing tea leaf. This version of the bulletproof drink has caffeine equivalent to that of half a standard coffee.

SERVES 1

2 matcha green tea bags
1 tablespoon butter
1–2 teaspoons MCT oil

1. Brew your green tea as per usual, then transfer to a blender, add the butter and MCT oil and blitz for 20 seconds, or until combined and frothy. Remove from the blender and serve.

Simple Turmeric Drink

Capsules and powders are fantastic as supplements, but if you can, always go down the path of wholefoods, as they contain many co-factors helpful in enzyme reactions. I've been eating raw turmeric and garlic for some time now and have even got my son into it.

SERVES 1

½ teaspoon grated fresh turmeric
¼ lemon
¼ teaspoon honey (optional)

1. Place the turmeric, lemon and honey (if using) in a mug. Top with boiling water and allow to steep for 2–3 minutes before drinking.

Nutty Choc Smoothie

Simple and delicious, adjust the quantities of cacao depending on how 'chocolatey' you like it.

SERVES 1

200 ml coconut milk or nut milk
handful of macadamias
2–3 tablespoons cacao powder
1 teaspoon vanilla bean powder or extract
pinch of sea salt
handful of ice

1. Throw all the ingredients in a blender and blitz for 20 seconds, or until smooth. Pour into a glass and serve.

The Anti-inflammatory Juice

Since my protocol is all about minimising the harmful effects of inflammation and protecting your mitochondria and gut, this recipe is a must-have!

SERVES 4

1 red pepper, *deseeded and roughly chopped*
400 g punnet of cherry tomatoes
2 cm knob of root ginger, *peeled and roughly chopped*
4 cm knob of fresh turmeric, *peeled and roughly chopped*
200 g kale leaves
1 small baby beetroot, *chopped*
500 ml cups water
2 tablespoons cold-pressed olive oil
handful of ice

1. Throw all the ingredients in a blender and blitz for 20–30 seconds, or until smooth. Pour into glasses and serve.

Gut Healer

Bone broth is packed full of probiotics, collagen, gelatine and glucosamine, making it therapeutic for our gut and soft tissues.

SERVES 1

400 ml Chicken Bone Broth (see recipe page 247)
1 teaspoon turmeric
pinch of cumin
pinch of sea salt
squeeze of lemon juice

1. Gently heat the broth in a saucepan and add the turmeric, cumin, salt and lemon juice. Allow to simmer for 2 minutes, then remove from the heat, adjust the seasonings and drink warm.

SAUCES, SPREADS AND SWEET TREATS

Aïoli

Aïoli is a great way to make your veggies more enticing. This is a basic recipe, but add spices to make it sexier, if you like. I'm a fan of adding 1 teaspoon of smokey paprika to mine.

MAKES ABOUT **500** ML

4 egg yolks
1 teaspoon Dijon mustard
1 garlic clove, *roughly chopped*
2 tablespoons lemon juice
400 ml olive oil
sea salt and freshly ground black pepper, to taste

1. In a food processor, combine the egg yolks, mustard, garlic and lemon juice. Blitz for 10 seconds. With the engine of the processor still running, slowly add the oil. Continue to add oil until you reach the required consistency. (It should resemble a mayonnaise. If too runny, add extra oil.) Season with salt and pepper. Store in a jar in the fridge and use as required.

Avocado Dressing

This is a great way to use up any ageing avocados and increase your intake of monounsaturated fats.

MAKES ABOUT **150** ML

1 ripe avocado
1 teaspoon Dijon mustard
1 tablespoon apple cider vinegar
1 tablespoon lemon juice
5–6 tablespoons olive oil
¼ bunch of fresh parsley
sea salt and freshly ground black pepper, to taste

1. Throw all the ingredients in a food processor or blender and blitz for 20–30 seconds, or until combined and smooth.

Homemade Herb Butter

I first came across homemade butter when I used to cook with the kids at my son's school, years ago. It's surprisingly easy to do and then to customise. It's also a good way to use up cream which is nearing its use-by date.

MAKES ABOUT 450 G

600 ml thick double cream
1 teaspoon fresh or dried oregano or thyme
sea salt, to taste

1. Pour the cream into a blender and blend at medium speed for 4–5 minutes, at which point in time the sound of the blender may change as the buttermilk begins to separate from the solid (the butter). Continue to blend for 30 seconds or so, until the solids form into a ball. Remove from the jug and place in a mixing bowl.
2. It's important at this stage to rid the butter of any excess buttermilk. Do this by kneading with your hands or pressing the butter against the bowl with the back of a wooden spoon until no more liquid comes out.
3. Transfer the butter to a mixing bowl, add the herbs and season with salt, mixing thoroughly.
4. Place the ball of butter on some baking paper, grab each corner and bring it together, then twist the corners tight. Store in the fridge.

Homemade Turmeric Butter

Once you get to grips with making your own butter, it'll open the door to customising your own.

MAKES ABOUT **450** G

600 ml thick double cream
1 teaspoon turmeric
sea salt, to taste

1. Make butter according to Homemade Herb Butter (see recipe page 271), Steps 1–2.
2. Transfer the butter to a mixing bowl, add the turmeric and season with salt, mixing thoroughly.
3. Place the ball of butter on some baking paper, grab each corner and bring it together, then twist the corners tight. Store in the fridge.

Macadamia Butter

Super-easy to make, this delicious nut butter forms the base of ice-creams and smoothies.

MAKES ABOUT **500** G

500 g raw macadamias

1. Throw all the macadamias in a high-performance blender and blitz for 30 seconds, or until the nuts have formed a smooth butter. Transfer to an airtight container.

Hazelnut Choc Spread

This sugar-free spread uses some of nature's superfoods. Use activated nuts, if you can, or raw nuts. It can be used as a spread or as the foundation for a smoothie or ice-cream.

MAKES ABOUT **245** G

125 g macadamia nuts
60 g cup Brazil nuts
60 g cup pecans
2 tablespoons cacao
1 tablespoon chia seeds

1. Throw all the ingredients in a blender and process for 1–2 minutes, or until smooth.

Gummie Bears

Perhaps not an obvious choice in a health book, especially as most of the gummie bears available on the market are unhealthy *and* aimed at kids. However, done simply, these can provide nourishment.

MAKES 12-15, DEPENDING ON MOULD SIZE

3½ tablespoons powdered gelatine
90 ml warm water
1½ tablespoons frozen raspberries
½ tablespoon stevia

1. Dissolve the gelatine in the warm water and let sit for 5 minutes.
2. Place a small saucepan over low heat and add the raspberries and stevia. Heat for 2–3 minutes. Remove from the hob and blitz with a stick blender until thoroughly processed.
3. Add the berry mixture to the gelatine and stir until fully combined. Pour into moulds and pop into the fridge or freezer in an airtight container. Remove when the gummies have fully set – about 45 minutes.

Keto Ice-cream

I'm not a massive ice-cream kinda guy, but this is a great recipe. It's inspired by Dave Asprey's bulletproof recipe. One caveat is, *don't* expect Häagen-Dazs, because this ice-cream tastes like dark rich chocolate – that is to say, not overly sweet, and maybe even a little bitter.

MAKES 1 BATCH

4 eggs
4 egg yolks
2 teaspoons vanilla extract
1 teaspoon apple cider vinegar or lime juice
3 tablespoons coconut oil
3 tablespoons MCT oil
100 g butter (room temperature)
60 g cacao
1 teaspoon honey
2 teaspoons toasted nuts (e.g. walnuts or macadamias), *chopped*

1. Throw all the ingredients except the nuts in a blender or food processor and blitz for 30–60 seconds on low–medium, or until the mixture is smooth. Transfer to a freezer-proof bowl.
2. Freeze for 1 hour, or until it reaches the consistency of ice-cream. Remove from the freezer 5–10 minutes before serving and top with the toasted nuts.

Sources

ARTICLES

Australian Institute of Health and Welfare, 'Australia's Health, 2016', https://www.aihw.gov.au/reports/statistics/behaviours-risk-factors/overweight-obesity/overview

Jim English and Ward Dean, 'Medium Chain Triglycerides: Beneficial Effects on Energy, Atherosclerosis and Ageing', *Nutrition Review*, 22 April 2013.

Tanjaniina Laukkanen, Hassan Khan, Francesco Zaccardi et al, 'Association Between Sauna Bathing and Fatal Cardiovascular and All-Cause Mortality Events', *JAMA Internal Medicine*, 4):542-548, April 2015.

SW Lazar, CE Kerr, RH Wasserman, JR Gray, DN Greve, MT Treadway, and B Fischl, 'Meditation Experience is Associated with Increased Cortical Thickness', *Neuroreport,* 16(17), 1893–1897, 2005.

E Luders, AW Toga, N Lepore and C Gaser, 'The Underlying Anatomical Correlates of Long-term Meditation: Larger Hippocampal and Frontal Volumes of Gray Matter', *Neuroimage,* 45(3), 672–678, 15 April, 2009.

Dr Joseph Mercola, 'Basic Introduction into Metabolic Mitochondrial Therapy', 2017. https://articles.mercola.com/sites/articles/archive/2017/05/21/metabolic-mitochondrial-therapy-introduction.aspx

Dr Joseph Mercola, 'Ketogenic Diet Often Better than Drugs in the Treatment for Epilepsy', 2017. https://articles.mercola.com/sites/articles/archive/2017/07/06/mmt-online-course.aspx

Dr Joseph Mercola, 'Ketogenic Diet Study Confirms Massive Anti-Inflammatory Affects', 2017. https://articles.mercola.com/sites/articles/archive/2017/10/09/ketogenic-diet-anti-inflammatory-effects.aspx

Dr Joseph Mercola, 'The Ketogenic Keys to Optimal Health', 2017.
https://articles.mercola.com/sites/articles/archive/2017/07/06/
mmt-online-course.aspx

Mark Sisson, 'Benefits of Keto', 10 June, 2017. https://www.marksdailyapple.
com/keto/benefits/

Mark Sisson, 'The Definitive Guide to Resistant Starch', 26 March, 2014.
https://www.marksdailyapple.com/the-definitive-guide-to-resistant-starch/

Mark Sisson, 'Putting out the Fire – Gut Flora and the Inflammatory Cycle',
4 May, 2010. https://www.marksdailyapple.com/gut-flora-inflammation/

Mark Sisson, 'Smart Fuel – Mushrooms', 19 August, 2014. https://www.
marksdailyapple.com/smart-fuel-mushrooms/

Taryn van Meygaarden, 'Bacteria and Obesity: Reviewing the Connection
between Gut Bacteria, Obesity, and Diet, *Holistic Performance Nutrition*,
2 August, 2017. http://www.holisticperformancenutrition.com/
articles--media/bacteria-and-obesity-reviewing-the-connection-between-
gut-bacteria-obesity-and-diet

Emily White, 'Why there is So Much More to it than Calories In and Calories
Out', *Holistic Performance Nutrition*, 14 August, 2017.
http://www.holisticperformancenutrition.com/articles--media/
why-there-is-so-much-more-to-it-than-just-calories-in-calories-out

BOOKS

Dr Loren Cordain, *The Paleo Diet*, John Wiley and Sons, New Jersey, 2011.

Giulia Enders, *Gut: The Inside Story of our Body's Most Under-rated Organ*,
Scribe, Melbourne, 2015.

Cliff Harvey, *The Carbohydrate Appropriate Diet*, Katoa Health Publishing,
Auckland, 2016.

Dr Joseph Mercola, *Fat for Fuel: A Revolutionary Diet to Combat Cancer, Boost
Brain Power, and Increase Your Energy*, Hay House, Carlsbad, 2017.

Michael Mosley, *The Clever Guts Diet*, Short Books Limited, London, 2017.

Michael Mosley, *The Fast Diet*, Short Books Limited, London, 2015.

Dr David Perlmutter, *Brain Maker: The Power of Gut Microbes to Heal and
Protect Your Brain – for Life*, Hodder & Stoughton, London, 2015.

Dr David Perlmutter, *Grain Brain: The Surprising Truth about Wheat, Carbs and
Sugar – Your Brain's Silent Killer*, Hodder & Stoughton, London, 2013.

Robb Wolf, *Wired to Eat: How to Rewire Your Appetite and Lose Weight for Good*,
Ebury, London, 2017.

VIDEOS AND PODCASTS

DR JOSEPH MERCOLA

'Dr Mercola interviews John Douillard', 2017. https://www.youtube.com/
watch?v=MaGAyp3QhBA

'Dr Mercola Interviews Dr Jason Fung', 2016. https://www.youtube.com/
watch?v=ETJ2YYOdBNE

'Dr Mercola interviews Gary Taubes', 2016. (https://www.youtube.com/
watch?v=Rfb5QjpdhNw)

DR DAVID PERLMUTTER

'Ketogenic Diet & Gut Bacteria', 2016. https://www.youtube.com/
watch?v=2hR9sD9eX-A&t=290s

'Keto Brain Hack – Ketogenic Diet Effects on the Brain' (with Dr Dominic
D'Agostino), 2017. https://www.youtube.com/watch?v=mpl2om711cM

GARY TAUBES

'The Case against Sugar', 6 January, 2017. https://www.youtube.com/
watch?v=2jla1ofRIiY&t=1521s

'The Joe Rogan Experience – Episode 904', 24 January, 2017. https://www.
youtube.com/watch?v=qoffswUVoxA&t=1086s

'Stem Talk, Episode 37 – Gary Taubes Discusses Low Carb Diets and Sheds
Light on the Hazards of Sugar, 9 May, 2017. https://www.youtube.com/
watch?v=FSmtbiAZXQ4&t=25s

'Why We Get Fat: The Diet/Weight Relationship, An Alternative Hypothesis',
21 November, 2014. https://www.youtube.com/watch?v=qEuIlQONcHw

DR TERRY WAHLS

TED Talk 'Minding your Mitochondria', 30 November, 2011. https://www.
youtube.com/watch?v=KLjgBLwH3Wc

ROBB WOLF

'Stem Talk – Episode 27: Robb Wolf discusses the Paleo Diet, Keto, Exercise,
Nicotine and Much More', 18 April, 2017. https://www.youtube.com/
watch?v=RkvqzoNvfGk

'Podcast 374, Robb Wolf interviews Mark Sisson – The Keto Reset Diet',
3 October, 2017. https://robbwolf.com/2017/10/03/episode-374-mark-sisson-
the-keto-reset-diet/

FURTHER READING

If some of the contents of this book seem confrontational and challenging, I urge you to do some further reading and research — try some of the sources I've listed above. The information isn't meant to scare you but rather open the door and spark a conversation with yourself. (Remind yourself that the status quo or conventional health guidelines have not served us well!) A very good place to start would be the websites of these researchers and doctors:

Dr Loren Cordain
thepaleodiet.com

Dr Joseph Mercola
www.mercola.com

Michael Mosley
cleverguts.com

Dr David Perlmutter
www.drperlmutter.com

Mark Sisson
www.marksdailyapple.com

Gary Taubes
garytaubes.com

Dr Terry Wahls
terrywahls.com

Robb Wolf
www.robbwolf.com

Acknowledgements

Thanks to everyone who has been incredibly supportive of this book. Writing a book is both hard work and ultimately revealing — so your support has been very much appreciated.

In my last book I acknowledged prominent commentators in the Australian health scene — I doff my cap to them again, and give additional thanks to researchers and doctors for disseminating important information about health. Thank you in particular to Dr Terry Wahls, author of *The Wahls Protocol, A Radical New Way to Treat All Chronic Autoimmune Conditions Using Paleo Principles*, for allowing me to tell her story in Chapter One, and Dr Loren Cordain for the use of his omega 6/omega 3 figures on page 96. In many ways I'm simply the conduit of information from these researchers — whom I believe to be sharing a credible health message addressing the problems associated with inflammation, gut health and cognitive function. So with this in mind, special thanks also to Dr David Perlmutter, Dr Cliff Harvey, Dr Dom D'Agostino, Dr Joseph Mercola and Robb Wolf. Without prominent researchers like you, this information would be much harder to come by.

Thank you to Bec and Tara for allowing me to tell their stories. Thanks also to Dr Giulia Enders, whose wonderful, entertaining yet informative book on the digestive system and gut health has been a great inspiration to me.

Thanks for reading — be healthy, be happy!

Scott

Scott Gooding is a passionate cook, health coach and personal trainer. He has worked with brands such as Whirlpool, Thrive, Huon Salmon, Body Science and Undivided Food Co which, along with his website www.scottgoodingproject.com has allowed him to share his true passion: to educate on healthy lifestyles through online information and inspiration, demos, presentations, classes and TV appearances. In 2013 he appeared on Channel 7's *My Kitchen Rules*, which enabled him to share his version of healthy food with Australians. He is also co-author of the bestselling Clean Living series of books and cookbooks.

Follow Scott online on:
scottgoodingproject.com
Facebook: Scott Gooding Project
Twitter: @scottgoodingpro
Instagram: @scottgoodingproject

Index

fruit 82

garlic 110
ghee 99
gluconeogenesis 76
gluten 35—7
gluten-free products 37
glycaemic, high 47, 78
glycation 36
gut health 18, 24
gut lining 25, 26—7, 28, 36

Hadza tribe 20
high fat diet 39, 42, 50
home-delivery 71—2
Hopkins, John 60
hydration 58, 117

immunity 18
immunogenic foods 23
inflammation 15, 24, 28, 36—7
insulin 6, 29, 30—2, 76
Inuit diet 42

keto diet
    classic 60—1, 132
    cyclic 132
    modified 61—2
    60-day Keto Diet Protocol 129—48
keto flu 56—7
ketogenic diet, benefits 40—2
ketone supplements 59, 110
ketones 43, 51, 53, 56, 86
ketosis 42—4, 49—50, 73, 131—2
Keyes, Ancel 6

labels and labelling 38, 66—7
lard 98
large intestine 17, 18
leaky gut 27
lemon 13
lion's mane 111—12, 144
lipid levels 133
low-fat foods 8
low FODMAP 45
lunch 68

macronutrients 10, 74
magnesium 58, 109
mammalian target of rapamycin
    (mTOR) 52, 77—8, 105
Marine Stewardship Council 95

meat
    alternative cuts 80
    grass-fed v grain-fed 81, 92—3
    organ derived 79—80
    portion size 78
medium-chain triglycerides (MCT) 58,
    93—4, 110
meditation and mindfulness 117—18,
    127
microbiome 18, 24
mitochondria 43, 55, 92, 94, 104
mouth 16
mucin 25, 28
multiple sclerosis 10—11, 124
    relapsing remitting 126

nutrition 3, 9, 102, 108

obesity 5—6, 33—4
oesophagus 16
olives and olive oil 97
omega 3 91—2, 94, 96
omega 6 91—2, 96
overcooking 13

paleo diet 46—8
pancreas 31
portion sizes 78
potassium 58
potato paradox, the 87
prebiotics 21, 28, 87
primal diet 48
processed foods 22—3
protein 46, 74—81
    cleanses and 76—7
    daily intake 75
    excess 75—8
    sources of 79—81
pulses and legumes 83

real food 5, 9—10, 23
Redgrave, Steve 32—3
reishi mushrooms 112—13, 144
resistant starch 87

saliva glands 16
salt 13, 57
satiety 78—9
saturated fats 4, 6
saunas 113—14
serotonin 18
serving sizes 67

RECIPES